Hospice/Palliative Care Training for Physicians: A Self-Study Program

UNIPAC Four: *Management of Selected Nonpain Symptoms in the Terminally Ill*

Authors

Porter Storey, M.D.
Clinical Associate Professor of Medicine and Assistant Professor of Family Medicine
Baylor College of Medicine

Consultant in Neuro-Oncology and Adjunct Assistant Professor of Medicine
University of Texas MD Anderson Cancer Center

Medical Director
The Hospice at the Texas Medical Center

Carol F. Knight, Ed.M.
Hospice Education Consultant

American Academy of Hospice and Palliative Medicine AAHPM

Copyright © 1996 by the American Academy of Hospice and Palliative Medicine
P.O. Box 14288
Gainesville, FL 32604-2288
Printed in U.S.A.   ISBN 1-889296-04-X

All rights reserved, including that of translation into other languages. No part of this publication may be reproduced or transmitted in any form or by any means, electronic or mechanical, including photocopying, recording, or any information storage and retrieval system, without permission in writing from the copyright holder.

Acknowledgments

The authors and the American Academy of Hospice and Palliative Medicine are deeply grateful to the following reviewers for their participation in the development of this UNIPAC. Their extensive comments and thoughtful suggestions greatly improved its contents.

We want to express special gratitude to the reviewers for coordinating local testing of the UNIPAC and to all the practicing physicians, fellows, residents, and medical students who participated in the field-testing.

Reviewers

Julia L. Smith, M.D.
  Assistant Professor of Oncology in Medicine
  University of Rochester Cancer Center

  Medical Director
  Genesee Region Home Care/Hospice
  Rochester, New York

John W. Finn, M.D.
  Clinical Assistant Professor
  Wayne State University School of Medicine
  Detroit, Michigan

  Medical Director
  Hospice of Michigan
  Southfield, Michigan

Eli N. Perencevich, D.O.
  Clinical Assistant Professor of Medicine
  Ohio State University

  Medical Director
  Hospice of Columbus
  Columbus, Ohio

Gerald H. Holman, M.D.
  Past Chief of Staff
  VA Medical Center

  Vice President for Medical Education
  Crown of Texas Hospice
  Amarillo, Texas

The American Academy of Hospice and Palliative Medicine's Self Study Training Program

The self-study program, *Hospice/Palliative Care Training for Physicians*, is under development by the American Academy of Hospice and Palliative Medicine and is made possible with federal funds from the National Cancer Institute's Cancer Education Grant Program, Grant # CA66771-02. The Academy recognizes a need for physician training materials on hospice/palliative care and has designed the self-study program to meet its own education goals, as well as those of the National Cancer Institute. The program consists of multiple modules, or UNIPACs, each of which follows the recommended format for self-instructional learning and includes behavioral objectives, a pretest, reading material, clinical situations for demonstrating knowledge application, a posttest and references.

UNIPACs currently being developed include (1) The Hospice/Palliative Approach to Caring for the Terminally Ill, (2) Psychological, Spiritual, and Physiological Aspects of Dying and Bereavement, (3) Assessment and Treatment of Pain in the Terminally Ill, (4) Management of Selected Nonpain Symptoms in the Terminally Ill, (5) Caring for the Terminally Ill: Communication and the Interdisciplinary Team Approach, and (6) Ethical and Legal Decision Making When Caring for the Terminally Ill.

Although the UNIPACs may be used by candidates when reviewing for the written examination of the American Board of Hospice and Palliative Medicine, they were not developed for that purpose. The Academy recommends that candidates also review basic information in the field of hospice/palliative medicine that can be found in a number of excellent resources.

The information presented and opinions expressed herein are those of the authors and do not necessarily represent the views of the sponsor or its parent agencies, the National Institutes of Health, the United States Public Health Service, the reviewers, or a consensus of the members of the American Academy of Hospice and Palliative Medicine. Any recommendations made by the authors must be weighed against the physician's own clinical judgment, based on but not limited to such factors as the patient's condition, benefits versus risks of suggested treatment, and comparison with recommendations of pharmaceutical compendia and other authorities.

The American Academy of Hospice and Palliative Medicine is accredited by the Accreditation Council for Continuing Medical Education (ACCME) to sponsor continuing medical education for physicians and therefore designates this CME activity for three (3) credit hours in Category 1 of the Physician's Recognition Award of the American Medical Association.

For information on the availability of specific UNIPACs and other Academy materials, please contact the American Academy of Hospice and Palliative Medicine at (352) 377-8900.

Management of Selected Nonpain Symptoms in the Terminally Ill

Table of Contents

About UNIPAC Four: *Management of Selected Nonpain Symptoms in the Terminally Ill* 1
    Introduction to the UNIPAC 2
    Pretest 4
    Behavioral Objectives 6
    Introduction to the Management of Selected Nonpain Symptoms 6

Anorexia and Dysphagia 9
    Introduction to Anorexia and Dysphagia 10
    Anorexia 10
    Dysphagia 14
    Clinical Situation Illustrating the Assessment
        and Treatment of Anorexia and Dysphagia 19

Dyspnea 25
    Introduction to Dyspnea 26
    Assessment and Treatment 26
    Clinical Situation Illustrating the Assessment
        and Treatment of Dyspnea 33

Nausea, Vomiting, and Bowel Obstruction 39
    Introduction to Nausea and Vomiting 40
    Pathophysiology of Vomiting 40
    Assessment and Treatment of Nausea and Vomiting 41
    Introduction to Bowel Obstruction 46
    Clinical Situation Illustrating the Assessment
        and Treatment of Nausea and Vomiting 49

Delirium and Terminal Restlessness 55
    Introduction to Delirium and Terminal Restlessness 56
    Delirium 56
    Restlessness 58
    Clinical Situation Illustrating the Assessment and
        Treatment of Delirium and Terminal Restlessness 61

Pretest Correct Responses 67

Posttest 69

References 77

Posttest Answer Sheet—Removable

Tables 4, 5 and 9 Reference Cards—Removable

Management of Selected Nonpain Symptoms in the Terminally Ill

Tables

Table 1	Symptom Prevalence in Patients with Cancer	7
Table 2	Reversible Causes of Anorexia	11
Table 3	Conditions that Interfere with Eating and Suggested Interventions	15
Table 4	Dysphagia: Causes and Treatments	16
Table 5	Specific Causes and Treatments for Dysphagia	28
Table 6	Pathophysiology of Vomiting	40
Table 7	Specific Measures for the Treatment of Nausea	43
Table 8	Suggested Antiemetics for Parenteral Use	45
Table 9	Pharmacological Treatment of Pain, Nausea, and Constipation Associated with Bowel Obstruction	48
Table 10	Common Causes of Delirium	57

About UNIPAC Four

Management of Selected Nonpain Symptoms in the Terminally Ill

- Introduction to the UNIPAC
  - Purpose
  - Recommended Procedure
  - Continuing Medical Education

- Pretest

- Behavioral Objectives

- Introduction to Management of Selected Nonpain Symptoms
  - Urgent Symptoms

About UNIPAC Four: *Management of Selected Nonpain Symptoms in the Terminally Ill*

Introduction to the UNIPAC

Purpose

A UNIPAC is a self-instructional training program. This UNIPAC describes nine nonpain symptoms commonly experienced by terminally ill patients, and presents specific, practical information designed to help physicians assess and manage each symptom. Clinical situations likely to be encountered on an almost daily basis are included to illustrate the application of specific management techniques.

The nine symptoms are combined into four symptom groups that are presented in the order in which they usually are experienced by terminally ill patients: (1) anorexia and dysphagia, (2) dyspnea, (3) nausea, vomiting, and bowel obstruction, and (4) terminal restlessness and delirium.

Three common nonpain symptoms—constipation, anxiety, and depression—are discussed in other UNIPACs. Because opioid therapy for pain control frequently causes or exacerbates constipation, the assessment and treatment of this commonly experienced nonpain symptom is included in *UNIPAC Three: Assessment and Treatment of Pain in the Terminally Ill*. Because anxiety and depression frequently are symptoms of troubling psychological and spiritual problems, including fear of abandonment and the search for hope and meaning, they are addressed in *UNIPAC Two: Psychological, Spiritual, and Physiological Aspects of Dying and Bereavement*. The pharmacologic management of anxiety and depression is often the least complicated aspect of their treatment.

Additional information is available from the American Academy of Hospice and Palliative Medicine, whose staff can direct you to physicians specializing in terminal care who are more than willing to share their experiences with the assessment and management of nonpain symptoms.

Recommended Procedure

To receive maximum benefit from this module the following procedure is recommended:

- Complete the pretest before reading the module.
- Review the behavioral objectives.
- Study each section and the accompanying clinical situation.
- Study the correct responses to the pretest.
- Complete the posttest by marking the correct answers on the answer sheet.

Continuing Medical Education

The American Academy of Hospice and Palliative Medicine designates this CME activity for three (3) credit hours in Category 1 of the Physician's Recognition Award of the American Medical Association. To receive CME credit for completing this UNIPAC, please follow the instructions on the Posttest Answer Sheet at the back of this publication.

About UNIPAC Four: *Management of Selected Nonpain Symptoms in the Terminally Ill*

Pretest

Before proceeding, please complete the following true/false items. The correct responses are included at the end of the UNIPAC.

	T	F
1. All anorexic terminally ill patients should be treated with appetite stimulants.		
2. Nasogastric tubes and/or diverting surgery are required to treat bowel obstructions in terminally ill patients.		
3. Acute onset helps distinguish delirium from dementia.		
4. When carefully titrated, hydrocodone (Hycodan), oxycodone, oral morphine, or hydromorphone (Dilaudid) can be effective treatments for dyspnea.		
5. Some antiemetics can be combined with morphine or hydromorphone (Dilaudid) in a subcutaneous (SC) infusion.		
6. Parenteral antiemetics such as haloperidol (Haldol) may be necessary to control severe cancer-related nausea.		
7. In some cases, artificial hydration/nutrition can contribute to a terminally ill patient's suffering.		
8. Drugs, sepsis, and electrolyte abnormalities are common causes of delirium.		
9. Anxiety, religious concerns, parenteral nutrition, and bronchospasm can contribute to dyspnea.		
10. Opioids are the first-choice agents for treating nonspecific dyspnea associated with terminal illness.		
11. Ordering megestrol (Megace) is an appropriate first step when treating anorexia.		
12. When dry mouth is a problem, ordering pilocarpine may be an effective initial step.		

	T	F

13. When treating nonspecific cancer-related dyspnea, naloxone (Narcan) should be ordered if the patient breathes <12/minute.

14. When starting opioid therapy for dyspnea in a 50-year-old male patient taking no pain medication, an appropriate order could be hydrocodone (Hycodan or Lortab) 5 mg q 4-6 hours.

15. When persistent nausea requires the use of SC antiemetics, metoclopramide (Reglan) can be combined with hydromorphone (Dilaudid) or morphine.

16. Ordering tranquilizers is likely to relieve nausea mediated by the vestibular apparatus.

17. When treating nausea associated with bowel obstruction, subcutaneous haloperidol (Haldol) 5-15 mg/day may be an appropriate order.

18. Treating mucositis with diluted viscous lidocaine may be an effective intervention for dysphagia.

19. Up to 30% of terminally ill patients experience delirium.

20. When attempts to reverse the causes of an agitated delirium fail or are inappropriate, an effective order might be haloperidol (Haldol) 2 mg PO or SC hourly until calm.

About UNIPAC Four: *Management of Selected Nonpain Symptoms in the Terminally Ill*

Behavioral Objectives

Upon completion of this UNIPAC, the physician should be able to demonstrate the ability to:

1. Assess for anorexia and dysphagia and provide effective interventions.
2. Assess for dyspnea and prescribe effective treatments.
3. Assess for nausea and vomiting and prescribe effective treatments.
4. Assess for bowel obstruction and prescribe the least invasive treatments.
5. Assess for delirium and terminal restlessness and prescribe effective interventions.

Introduction to the Management of Selected Nonpain Symptoms

Terminally ill patients frequently experience distressing nonpain symptoms during the last months of life. Although the assessment and management of pain has received more attention, nonpain symptoms can be just as troubling for both dying patients and practitioners.

The sometimes complicated pathophysiology of nonpain symptoms coupled with limited data about their effective treatment may present management challenges for even the most experienced practitioner. Despite these problems, successful treatment of nonpain symptoms usually is possible and contributes greatly to the patient's quality of life. When the underlying disease process cannot be cured, all symptoms become magnified and demand rapid and skilled control.[1]

As with the treatment of pain, completing a thorough history and physical is the most important first step when treating nonpain symptoms. In addition, the following are necessary for managing nonpain symptoms:

- Careful assessment of each symptom
- Use of effective doses of medication
- Patient and family education
- Involvement of the entire interdisciplinary team
- Continual reassessment

Table 1 lists symptoms commonly experienced by terminally ill cancer patients.

Table 1

Symptom Prevalence in Patients with Cancer [2,3]

Symptom	Prevalence (as a percentage)		
	Edmonton Palliative Care Service, Canada	St. Christopher's Hospice, U.K.	Memorial Sloan-Kettering Cancer Center, U.S.A.
Asthenia	90%	91%	74%
Anorexia	85	76	44
Pain	76	62	64
Nausea	68	44	44
Constipation	65	51	35
Sedation/confusion	60	N/A	60
Dyspnea	12	51	24

Urgent Symptoms

During the assessment process, clinicians should maintain a high index of suspicion for symptoms such as the following that may require aggressive management due to their severe impact on the patient's and family's quality of life:

- Fracture
- Seizure
- Spinal cord compression
- Hypercalcemia
- Increased intracranial pressure
- Superior vena cava syndrome

In hospice/palliative care settings, treating distressing symptoms is always necessary but, in many cases, treating underlying diseases may not be appropriate. Analgesics and adjuvant drugs such as steroids should be used immediately to control symptoms, but the likely benefits and burdens of other therapies, in particular disease-modifying therapies such as radiation and chemotherapy, require careful evaluation.

In most cases, moribund patients should receive only symptomatic treatment; however, alert and ambulatory patients may have more choices. In some cases, spinal cord compression and superior vena cava obstruction l signal the onset of conditions whose rapid downhill course can be alleviated

About UNIPAC Four: *Management of Selected Nonpain Symptoms in the Terminally Ill*

with early treatment. However, before initiating treatment, the physician, patient/surrogate, and family should discuss the following:

- The diagnostic and therapeutic procedures that may be required and their effects on the patient
- The patient's condition and the likely benefits and burdens of proposed treatments, including their cost
- Alternative methods of palliating these symptoms

Patients and families will greatly appreciate the physician's caring interest, guidance, and assistance with understanding various treatment options. Because the acute management of urgent symptoms is beyond the scope of this UNIPAC, clinicians should refer to other resources, including the *Oxford Textbook of Palliative Medicine* by Doyle, Hanks, and MacDonald, which is published by Oxford University Press.

Anorexia and Dysphagia

- Introduction to Anorexia and Dysphagia

- Anorexia
  - Assessment and Treatment
  - Physical Conditions that Interfere with Appetite
  - Psychosocial Issues that Interfere with Appetite
  - Appetite Stimulants
  - Artificial Nutrition
    - Hospice/Palliative Care Literature
    - Consider Practical Issues

- Dysphagia
  - Conditions that Interfere with Eating and Suggested Interventions
  - Causes and Treatments for Dysphagia
  - Irreversible Dysphagia

- Clinical Situation Illustrating the Assessment and Treatment of Anorexia and Dysphagia

Introduction to Anorexia and Dysphagia

Anorexia and dysphagia are common, interrelated symptoms experienced by most terminally ill patients. Both symptoms, with their associated progressive cachexia, are particularly distressing to patients and their families because lack of appetite and progressive weight loss are associated with deteriorating health and approaching death.

Anorexia

Assessment and Treatment

Anorexia, or loss of appetite for food, is a common complication of advanced cancer, HIV, and other terminal illnesses. Its causes are multiple and may include endogenous cytokines, metabolic disturbances, and infections as well as other reversible physical and psychosocial problems.[4] Before treating anorexia, the practitioner should first complete a careful history and physical examination with special emphasis on treatable physical conditions and psychosocial issues that interfere with appetite.

Physical Conditions that Interfere with Appetite

Although lack of interest in food is a common symptom of depression, the anorexia of advanced disease is more often caused by treatable physical symptoms and difficulties with the mechanical process of eating. The practitioner first should assess and aggressively treat any complicating treatable physical conditions that may be interfering with appetite, such as unrelieved pain, a dry or painful mouth, difficulty swallowing, nausea, and constipation. When treating anorexia, consider the reversible factors listed in Table 2.

Psychosocial Issues that Interfere with Appetite

In an effort to forestall the approaching death of a loved one, family members may respond to a terminally ill patient's loss of appetite and progressive cachexia by focusing their concerns on the patient's eating habits. Family members may inadvertently precipitate food-related conflicts by continuing to prepare unwanted food and then feeling angry and rejected when lovingly prepared meals are refused. Such conflicts can occur even when the patient accepts decreased appetite as part of the dying process.

Table 2

	Reversible Causes of Anorexia	
A	Aches and pains	See *UNIPAC Three: Assessment and Treatment of Pain*
N	Nausea and gastrointestinal dysfunction	See page 40
O	Oral candidiasis	See page 16
R	Reactive (or organic) depression	In *UNIPAC Two*, see *Depression*
E	Evacuation problems (constipation, retention)	In *UNIPAC Three*, see *Adverse Side Effects*
X	Xerostomia (dry mouth)	See page 16
I	Iatrogenic (radiation, chemotherapy, or drugs)	See page 16
A	Acid-related problems (gastritis, peptic ulcers)	Consider cimetidine or other H_2 blocking agents. Protect patients at risk for ulcers who require a non-steroidal anti-inflammatory drug (NSAID) with misoprostol (Cytotec)

For more information, see pages 15-17.

When appropriate, physicians can help defuse food-related conflicts by offering nonspecific measures such as the following:

- Provide patient and family education about the natural progression of cancer and its effects on appetite.
  - Anorexia is part of the disease process.
  - The patient is not starving to death.
  - Forced feeding may cause discomfort.
  - Artificial feeding usually does not prolong life and may shorten it.
  - Patients can live comfortably for a long time on very little food.

- Provide sensible dietary advice.
  - Involve the patient in menu planning.
  - Offer small portions of the patient's favorite foods.
  - Unless the patient requests them, avoid foods with strong odors.
  - Offer easy-to-swallow foods, such as semi-liquids, puddings, or soft or puréed foods.
- Help family members identify alternative methods of expressing their love for the patient. Interactions that focus on something other than eating can be helpful, for instance looking at family photograph albums, listening to music together, reading aloud, and giving gentle massages.

Appetite Stimulants

Pharmacological stimulation of appetite is not always successful, but some patients may benefit from appetite stimulants. If the interventions suggested in Table 3 on page 15 do not relieve anorexia, a short trial of appetite stimulants may be appropriate.

Key Point: If the patient experiences no benefits within a week, either increase the dose or discontinue the medication to avoid unnecessary side effects and expense.

When appetite stimulants are appropriate, consider:

- **Megestrol**—80-200 mg 3-4 times a day can be effective for patients with cancer[5] or HIV.[6]
- **Prednisone**—10-20 mg 1-2 times a day, *or* dexamethasone 2-4 mg, 1-2 times a day. Corticosteroids are helpful for patients who have a shorter prognosis or other indications for steroid use, such as bronchospasm or bone pain.
- **Dronabinol (Marinol)**—2.5-5 mg 2-3 times a day, especially for patients with HIV who cannot tolerate megestrol.[7]

Artificial Nutrition

Before initiating oral or parenteral tube feedings for the treatment of anorexia, the physician should discuss the following information so patients and families will not have unrealistic expectations about the likely effects of treatment.

Key Point: The physician's kind and informed concern, coupled with aggressive treatment of other symptoms, will make this news easier to accept.

Hospice/Palliative Care Literature

The hospice/palliative care literature suggests the following:

- Tube feedings and forced feedings in terminally ill patients have never been shown to prolong life. They are sometimes associated with an increase in the basal metabolic rate.[8]

- Total parenteral nutrition (TPN) for cancer chemotherapy patients has been shown by meta-analysis of 12 randomized trials to be associated with **decreased** survival, **decreased** response to chemotherapy, and an **increased** rate of infection. The American College of Physicians could not identify any subgroup in which such treatment appeared to be of benefit.[9] TPN for patients with HIV mostly increases body fat and has not been shown to improve survival.[10]

- In one teaching hospital, it was observed that survival times from the issuance of "do not resuscitate" orders to death were significantly longer among cancer patients who did not receive IV fluids than among those who did.[11]

- Nasogastric or gastrostomy tube feedings, especially in the elderly, are associated with a high incidence of aspiration pneumonia, self-extubation, use of restraints, and symptoms such as nausea, rattling respiratory secretions, and diarrhea.[12]

- The observations of many experienced hospice professionals indicate that artificial nutrition does not increase the comfort of terminally ill patients.[13, 14, 15, 16] Parenteral hydration by hypodermoclysis may have a role in the treatment of intractable thirst or delirium in some patients.

Consider Practical Issues

When making decisions about artificial nutrition, family members also may want to consider practical issues such as the following:

- Nasogastric tubes are uncomfortable and unattractive. Gastrostomy tubes require surgery, a procedure that entails some risk and discomfort.

- The fragile veins of most terminally ill patients make it difficult to insert an intravenous needle, and IV sites may need to be changed frequently.

- Artificial nutrition and hydration may increase secretions, ascites, or effusions, which then require additional treatment.

Dysphagia

Terminally ill patients, in particular those with cancer or acquired immune deficiency syndrome (AIDS), have significant and specific oral care needs that must be addressed in the treatment and prevention of dysphagia. Because conservative management can ameliorate dysphagia in a majority of patients with terminal cancer, a comprehensive, interdisciplinary treatment plan should emphasize good oral hygiene and other specific measures as appropriate.

Conditions that Interfere with Eating and Suggested Interventions

Table 3 lists some of the common conditions that interfere with eating and includes suggestions for possible interventions. When dysphagia initially presents as difficulty swallowing solids and then progresses to difficulty swallowing liquids, the cause is often obstructing lesions. When dysphagia for solids and liquids occurs almost simultaneously, neuromuscular disorders are frequently the cause.

Causes and Treatments for Dysphagia

Table 4 lists some of the common causes of dysphagia and includes suggested treatments.

Irreversible Dysphagia

When dysphagia is due to esophageal obstruction, or when it is irreversible or progressive, the practitioner and the interdisciplinary team should consider whether or not the patient is a suitable candidate for more invasive measures such as the following:

- Surgical resection or laser ablation of an obstructing lesion
- Palliative radiation therapy
- Placement of an esophageal stent

In most cases, these procedures are neither practical nor desired. In some instances (e.g., mechanical obstruction with complaints of hunger), a nasogastric or gastrostomy tube or hypodermoclysis may provide more benefits than burdens. See *Artificial Nutrition* on page 12.

Helping the family cope with feelings of anxiety and guilt about the patient's low intake may be the most important intervention. As always, teamwork is essential.

Table 3

Conditions that Interfere with Eating and Suggested Interventions

Condition	Intervention
Dentures that fit poorly	• Adjust dentures or get new dentures. • Offer puréed foods.
Poor dental hygiene	• Encourage brushing and flossing 2-3 times a day.
Taste disorders	• Treat sinusitis or other infections. • Provide supplemental vitamins, zinc, and other minerals.
Weakness or neuromuscular problems	• Offer soft or pureed foods. • Cut food into bite-sized pieces. • Provide small frequent meals. • Moisten food with gravy, sauce, sour cream, or mayonnaise. • Avoid hard, dry, or sticky foods. • Assist to upright position and stabilize head. • Use aids for easier drinking and eating, i.e., a drinking glass with a cut-out for the nose. • Use crushed, liquid, or rectal suppository forms of medication. • Encourage the patient to chew thoroughly and to remain upright for 15 minutes after eating.
Stress and tension	• Provide a calm, unhurried environment.

Table 4

Dysphagia: Causes and Treatments	
Condition	**Consider these treatments**
Dry mouth caused by radiation	• Pilocarpine 5-10 mg three times per day (watch for troublesome respiratory secretions or diarrhea)[17] • Saliva substitute every 1-2 hours • Pilocarpine + saliva substitute
Dryness caused by drugs	• Reduce dosage if possible. • Change the medication, e.g., use metoclopramide (Reglan) or haloperidol (Haldol) instead of prochlorperazine (Compazine) or chlorpromazine (Thorazine). Use doxepin (Sinequan) or trazodone (Desyrel) instead of amitriptyline (Elavil). • Apply fluoride to prevent dental damage.
Oral candidiasis	• Nystatin suspension • Clotrimazole (Mycelex) 10 mg troches, one troche dissolved in mouth five times daily. (Patient compliance may be a problem when dry mouth is also present.) For persistent problems: • Ketoconazole (Nizoral), 200 mg 1-2 tablets daily for 10-14 days • Fluconazole (Diflucan) 100 mg 1-2 times daily for 10-14 days
Bacterial infection	• The most common cause is periodontal disease. Consider adequate oral hygiene and an antibiotic.
Viral infection	• Acyclovir (Zovirax) 400 mg five times daily for 7-10 days

Table 4 *(continued from previous page)*

Condition	Consider these treatments
Reflux esophagitis	• Cimetidine (Tagamet), 300 mg every 6 hours, or other H_2 blocking agent • Place patient in more upright position by putting bricks under the head of the bed • Omeprazole (Prilosec) 20 mg daily

Mucosal damage from other causes[18]	• Peridex® or oral lavage with 1 teaspoon of sodium bicarbonate (baking soda) to 1 quart of water
	• Combination mouthwash utilizing two to three of the following:
	  a) diphenhydramine (Benadryl)
	  b) viscous xylocaine
	  c) Maalox or Kaopectate
	  d) nystatin
	  e) tetracycline
	  f) hydrocortisone
	• Xylocaine (Lidocaine) viscous 2%, 2-5 milliliters every 4-8 hours (can be diluted or flavored if desired). Can cause aspiration if used before meals.
	• Sucralfate (Carafate) suspension 5 milliliters swish and swallow 3-4 times daily
	• Parenteral opioids
	• Thalidomide 200 mg daily (known to cause malformations in infants born to women taking this drug)

Dryness caused by systemic dehydration	• Increase liquid intake by mouth if possible— try frozen juice or flavored ices. • Ice chips, atomizer, and sips of water. (As death approaches, encouraging family members to keep the patient's mouth moist with a few drops of water from a syringe or with a moist sponge stick may relieve dry mouth better than parenteral fluids and involves the family in the patient's care.)[19]

Clinical Situation Illustrating the Assessment of Anorexia and Dysphagia

Clinical Situation: Huong and Kim and their Grown Children

Huong is a 67-year-old man with colon cancer who is referred for hospice/palliative care. When the hospice/palliative care team first visits with Huong and his family, the primary complaint voiced by Huong's family concerns Huong's lack of appetite. Huong's wife, Kim, and his adult children are extremely upset because Huong is not eating. They are particularly worried about his lack of appetite because the dietitian at a regional cancer center told them that unless Huong swallowed six cans of nutritional supplement every day, he would need to have a tube put down his nose so food could be poured into his stomach.

Huong says he just doesn't feel like eating. He says the supplements are not to his liking and he does not want a tube in his nose. His principal complaints are discomfort in his abdomen and increasing weakness.

Question One

At this point, which of the following is the most appropriate intervention?

[A] Insert a nasogastric tube for delivery of artificial nutrition.

[B] Complete a history and physical.

[C] Insert a central venous catheter for total parenteral nutrition (TPN).

[D] Reassure the family that Huong's lack of appetite is normal.

[E] Order slow-release morphine 30 mg a day for abdominal pain.

Correct Response and Analysis

The correct response is B. More information is needed before making any decisions about interventions. The simple maneuver of completing a history and physical is most likely to reveal information about Huong's discomfort and lack of appetite, and will cause him the least amount of physical and financial distress. Although family reassurance and education about Huong's lack of appetite is likely to be an appropriate intervention in the near future, offering it now is premature because treatable causes of his lack of appetite may be revealed.

The Case Continues

A detailed history reveals that Huong was diagnosed with colon cancer one year ago and has documented metastases to his liver. He has had chemotherapy, but when the disease began to progress, the oncologist indicated Huong was no longer a candidate for further treatment. For the past several months Huong has had fluid drawn off his abdomen (paracentesis) approximately once a month. His medication is acetaminophen with codeine 30 mg (Tylenol #3) 1 tablet four times a day, which provides moderate pain relief. Huong is eating a few bites of soft food four times a day; however, despite his very limited intake, his weight has decreased only 10 pounds over the past 30 days due to his increased ascites. Huong drinks fluids with his meals and sips water throughout the day. He has not had a bowel movement for 6 days.

The physical exam reveals a blood pressure of 90 over 60, a pulse of 100, and regular respirations at 18 per minute. Huong's chest is clear to auscultation, his heart has a rapid but regular rate, and his abdomen is mildly distended with an enlarged, palpable liver in the right upper quadrant and moderate ascites. Some tenderness is present in the lower quadrants. Huong's extremities show some muscle wasting, and he has 2 + edema in his ankles. An examination of his oral mucosa reveals white patches on the palate, and he admits to some discomfort on swallowing. A rectal exam reveals a large amount of soft stool. Huong is in no apparent acute distress but is so weak he can barely transfer himself from his bed to the bedside commode.

Question Two

At this point, which two of the following are the most appropriate interventions?

[A] Order prednisone 20 mg three times a day to stimulate appetite.

[B] Order megestrol (Megace) 200 mg four times a day to stimulate appetite.

[C] Encourage feedings six times a day with an accurate calorie count.

[D] Order nystatin suspension (Mycostatin) 4 cc four times a day for oral candidiasis and senna (Senokot) 5 mg three times a day for constipation.

[E] Provide family education about Huong's cancer and its probable effects on his appetite.

Correct Response and Analysis

The correct responses are D and E. In addition to the effects of his liver metastases, oral candidiasis and constipation are the most likely contributing causes of Huong's lack of appetite. Both are common problems that should be treated aggressively with very specific remedies. Even though nystatin (Mycostatin) is effective only about half the time, it is an appropriate first choice in this situation. Ketoconazole (Nizoral), which is a more potent treatment, could have an adverse effect on the liver and Huong's liver is already compromised. Fluconazole (Diflucan) 100 mg daily is an appropriate but expensive second choice if the nystatin (Mycostatin) proves to be ineffective after a one-week trial. Patient and family education about Huong's cancer and its effects on his appetite are now appropriate.

The Case Continues

Huong becomes much more comfortable after his constipation and oral thrush are addressed. His pain is now controlled with oxycodone and acetaminophen (Percocet) 1 tablet every 4 hours, and an additional tablet one to two times a day for breakthrough pain. Huong's food intake increases slightly but not to his family's satisfaction. The physician, nurse, and social worker continue to address the family's concerns about Huong's illness, his progressive deterioration, and his continuing lack of appetite.

On reevaluation, Huong's pain, constipation, and oral candidiasis are under much better control. Family stress has subsided somewhat as a result of the team's education and supportive counseling interventions. A physical exam reveals a less distended and less tender abdomen, a large palpable mass in the right upper quadrant, and very few bowel sounds. Huong complains of mild nausea, particularly when smelling food, and says he feels full after eating just a few bites of food.

On the advice of the hospice nurse, the family avoids serving foods with strong odors, and the physician prescribes metoclopramide (Reglan) 10 mg four times a day before meals to reduce nausea and improve gastric emptying. This intervention controls Huong's nausea. Although Huong is silent when asked about his appetite, his low intake is a continuing family complaint. A reevaluation finds Huong somewhat thinner. His pain, oral thrush, nausea, and constipation are adequately controlled. He has increased bowel sounds and an enlarging liver in the right upper quadrant.

Anorexia and Dysphagia

Question Three

At this point, which two of the following are the most appropriate interventions?

[A] Continue patient and family education about the natural history of cancer and its effects on appetite to relieve the anxiety and guilt associated with reduced appetite.

[B] Order prednisone 20 mg daily to stimulate appetite.

[C] Order megestrol (Megace) 200 mg four times a day to stimulate appetite.

[D] Order lorazepam 1 mg four times a day to reduce patient anxiety.

[E] Order chlorpromazine (Thorazine) 100 mg at bedtime to reduce patient anxiety.

Correct Response and Analysis

Correct responses are A and either B or C. A is correct because it is appropriate to continue patient and family education interventions concerning the natural progression of cancer and its effects on appetite. B or C is correct because a trial course of an appetite stimulant is appropriate when lack of appetite continues to be the primary complaint after specific causes of anorexia have been treated and after patient guilt and family stress about lack of appetite have been addressed.

The Case Continues

A trial course of an appetite stimulant is started for a week or so, but swallowing the necessary number of tablets becomes a burden for Huong, and he and his family are not sure the treatment is making any difference in his intake; on some days he eats a little more, but on others he eats less.

Members of the interdisciplinary team note Huong's abdication of his decision-making authority to his family and discuss at length the issue of "Whose problem is this?" The team tries to minimize the adverse effects of the family's preoccupation with Huong's appetite by reinforcing education and supportive counseling interventions. Once again, family members are reassured that artificial nutrition and hydration will not increase Huong's length of life and, with their concurrence, the appetite stimulant is discontinued. Huong's family is relieved to hear they are doing everything possible and want to remain involved with his care.

When Huong is no longer able to swallow his oxycodone and acetaminophen (Percocet) tablets, he is switched to morphine concentrate and metoclopramide (Reglan) syrup, which control his pain and nausea, and to bisacodyl suppositories, which control his constipation. As Huong's condition deteriorates, his mental status diminishes and he requires more frequent visits from the hospice nurse and the home health aide. A Foley catheter is inserted and the physician orders chlorpromazine (Thorazine) 50 mg by tablets or rectal suppository at bedtime to help Huong and his family rest during the night.

Once again, the family consults with the hospice physician about Huong's poor oral intake. On reevaluation Huong is barely responsive to tactile and verbal stimuli. He can open his eyes, and he can respond to questions and indicate he is not experiencing pain. Huong's abdominal tumor is now quite large and he has severe muscle wasting. His chest exam shows decreased breath sounds in both bases. His constipation remains controlled with bisacodyl suppositories. His skin remains in good condition due to the excellent and loving care he is receiving from his family and the hospice team, but he has little skin turgor and has "tenting" of the skin folds and other signs of dehydration.

Question Four

At this point, which two of the following are the most appropriate interventions?

[A] Insert a nasogastric feeding tube for artificial nutrition.

[B] Start an IV with D5 half normal saline at 30 cc/hour for intravenous hydration.

[C] Offer dexamethasone 4 mg SC three times a day to stimulate appetite.

[D] Discontinue the morphine and metoclopramide (Reglan) to improve Huong's mental status.

[E] Provide family support and education about Huong's approaching death from colon cancer, and remind the family that keeping his mouth moist is a comforting and appropriate intervention they can provide.

Correct Response and Analysis

The correct response is E. Continued support by the entire hospice team is necessary as the patient's condition deteriorates and family members question whether or not they are doing everything they can to care for Huong. At this point, keeping Huong's mouth moist with a few drops of water from a syringe or a moistened sponge stick (Toothette) is the most effective intervention. The use of saline drops for the eyes and petroleum jelly on his lips is also appropriate. The other responses are incorrect. At this time, artificial nutrition and hydration are likely to increase Huong's discomfort by exacerbating his ascites and edema. A course of an appetite stimulant already has been tried with no success. Huong's decreased mental status is the result of the normal dying process, and discontinuing the morphine and metoclopramide (Reglan) will result only in a return of pain and nausea.

The Case Concludes

The team increases the frequency of its visits and Huong dies comfortably 2 days later. Family members are grateful for the intervention of the physician and the hospice team, and they appreciate the team's efforts to respond to their concerns.

Dyspnea

- Introduction to Dyspnea
- Assessment and Treatment
  - Specific Causes and Treatments for Dyspnea
  - General Treatment Measures for Dyspnea
  - Opioid Therapy
    - Mild Dyspnea
    - Severe Dyspnea or Dyspnea Being Treated with Weak Opioids
    - Severe Anxiety or Dyspnea Being Treated with Strong Opioids
  - Use of Oxygen
  - Use of Naloxone (Narcan)
  - Continual Reassessment
  - Terminal Sedation
- Clinical Situation Illustrating the Assessment and Treatment of Dyspnea

Introduction to Dyspnea

Dyspnea can be defined as an uncomfortable awareness of breathing. The treatment of dyspnea, or breathlessness, presents challenges for the practitioner because dyspnea, like pain, is a subjective sensation with a complicated pathophysiology that is affected by physical, psychological, social, and spiritual factors. The involvement of the entire interdisciplinary team is essential for treating dyspnea effectively.

Estimates of the prevalence of dyspnea among terminally ill patients vary from 12% to 74%; however, dyspnea is most common in patients with lung cancer, and it tends to worsen as death approaches.[20]

Patients describe dyspnea in different ways, including the following:

- Cannot get enough air
- Air does not go all the way down
- Smothering feeling in the chest
- Tightness in the chest
- Fatigue in the chest
- Choking sensation
- Feeling a need to gasp or pant
- Extreme fear of suffocation
- Harder to breathe in than to breathe out

Remember that respiratory effort and dyspnea are not the same—the patient may report substantial relief of dyspnea from opioids without a change in respiratory rate.

Assessment and Treatment

A careful history and physical are necessary to identify the causes of dyspnea, many of which can be treated. Breathlessness (dyspnea) as a symptom should be distinguished from symptoms such as the following, which do not necessarily indicate subjective distress:

- Tachypnea (rapid breathing)
- Hyperpnea (excessively deep breathing)
  - in acidosis
  - altered respiratory pattern with CNS lesion

In hospice/palliative care, the use of pulmonary function tests, arterial blood gases, echocardiography, and pulmonary angiography are rarely needed. The following general principles for treating dyspnea are the same as for any other hospice/palliative care intervention:

- Determine and treat the underlying cause whenever possible *and* reasonable for the patient.

- Consider the benefits and burdens of each specific treatment in terms of the prognosis and potential for improved quality of life for each patient.
- Discuss all treatment options (including symptom relief only) with the patient and family, and assist them with making these difficult decisions.

Specific Causes and Treatments

In the terminally ill population, dyspnea often has multiple etiologies. During the history and physical, it is important to try to establish the primary cause of dyspnea because each specific cause requires a different treatment. Look carefully for the causes listed in Table 5, and remember that anxiety is almost always a factor; it is both a cause and an effect of dyspnea. If the history and physical are inconclusive, additional tests to establish the primary cause of dyspnea may be warranted **IF:**

- The patient's prognosis is longer than a week or two.
- Attempts at symptomatic treatment are unsuccessful.
- Test results will alter the management of the patient in ways that are likely to result in more benefit than burden for the patient.

Table 5 lists some of the most common causes of dyspnea and includes suggested treatments.

General Treatment Measures for Dyspnea

General treatment measures for dyspnea include the following:

- Reduce the need for exertion and arrange for readily available help.
- Reposition the patient, usually to a more upright position or with the compromised lung down.
- Address skin care of the buttocks if the patient cannot stand or turn.
- Improve air circulation.
  - Provide a draft—use fans, open windows.
  - Adjust humidity with humidifier or air conditioner.
- Address anxiety and provide reassurance.
  - Discuss need for companionship and spiritual support. Isolation and spiritual concerns can exacerbate symptoms.
  - Discuss the meaning of symptoms and other patient/family concerns.
  - Anticipate and rehearse with the patient/family their responses when symptoms worsen.

(continued on page 29)

Table 5

Specific Causes and Treatments for Dyspnea

B **Bronchospasm**—If present, consider nebulized albuterol and/or oral steroids; if not present, consider lowering doses of theophylline and adrenergic agents to reduce any tremor and anxiety that often exacerbate dyspnea.

R **Rales**—If volume overload is present, reduce artificial feeding or stop IV fluids. Diuretics are occasionally needed. If pneumonia seems likely, decide whether an antibiotic will rehabilitate the patient or just prolong the dying process. Patient and family participation in this decision is essential.

E **Effusions**—Thoracentesis can be effective, but if the effusion recurs and the patient is ambulatory, consider chest tube pleurodesis to prevent recurrent lung collapse. If the patient is close to death, palliate the dyspnea with opioids and loving kindness.

A **Airway obstruction**—Make sure tracheostomy appliances are cleaned regularly. If aspiration of food is likely, purée solids and thicken liquids with cornstarch or "Thick-it," and instruct the family in positioning the patient during feeding and suctioning if necessary.

T **Thick secretions**—If the cough reflex is still strong, loosen secretions with nebulized saline. If the cough is weak, dry secretions with hyoscyamine (Levsin) 0.125 mg PO or SL q 8 hours or Transderm Scop 1-3 patches every 3 days, or add glycopyrrolate (Robinul) 0.4-1.0 mg per day to a subcutaneous infusion or by SC or IV bolus 0.2 mg q 3 hours prn. These drugs also reduce the so-called "death rattle."

H **Hemoglobin low**—A blood transfusion may add energy and reduce dyspnea for a few weeks.[21] More often, hemorrhage or marrow failure are part of the dying process and are best palliated with opioids and loving kindness.

A **Anxiety**—Sitting upright, using a bedside fan, listening to calming music, and practicing relaxation techniques can be extremely effective, as can skillful counseling and the presence of a calming physician. Dyspnea exacerbates normal fears and anxiety, so treat it with opioids first, then try a benzodiazepine if needed. If the opioid dose is limited by drowsiness, reduce the benzodiazepine and increase the opioid.

I **Interpersonal issues**—Social and financial problems contribute to dyspnea. Counseling and interaction with social workers and other members of the interdisciplinary team may bring relief. When family relationships exacerbate the problem, a few days spent in a peaceful, homelike hospice inpatient unit may help relieve the patient's symptoms.

R **Religious concerns**—Although faith or an experience of the transcendent can bring profound comfort, some religious beliefs, such as "God is punishing me" or "God will heal me if I have enough faith," can precipitate dyspnea and/or exacerbate its symptoms. Take time to listen with full attention and presence. Help the patient explore ways to reconnect with God, the cosmos, or the deepest parts of the self. Coordinate treatment with the patient's spiritual adviser, chaplain, counselor, other health care professionals, and family members.

(continued from page 27)

– Identify situational components, i.e., what triggers the dyspnea attack.

– Teach behavioral interventions such as relaxation and hypnosis.

• Discuss any patient/family/staff concerns about using opioids for dyspnea.

Opioid Therapy

When no treatable etiology can be identified or when the treatments already mentioned do not completely alleviate distressing symptoms, opioids are the first-choice agents for treating dyspnea because they suppress respiratory awareness so effectively. When individually titrated, opioids have been shown repeatedly to be safe and effective in the treatment of dyspnea caused by cancer.[22] In COPD patients, opioids decrease breathlessness and increase exercise tolerance with decreased ventilation.[23]

To treat dyspnea, order the same opioids on the same schedules as those prescribed for pain and increase the dose by 30% to 50% every 4-12 hours until the patient is comfortable.

Mild Dyspnea

For mild dyspnea in patients taking no pain medications, begin with low doses of an opioid such as one of the following:

• **Hydrocodone** (Hycodan or Lortab)— 5 mg tab q 4 hours with a booster dose of 5 mg every 2 hours prn

• **Acetaminophen with codeine**— (Tylenol #3)—30 mg (1 tab) q 4 hours with a booster dose of 30 mg every 2 hours prn

Children and the elderly may require lower doses, so break tablets in half or consider hydrocodone syrup 1-3 ml q 4 hours with booster doses of the full 4-hour dose prn.

Severe Dyspnea or Dyspnea Being Treated with Weak Opioids

For severe dyspnea in patients who are taking no pain medication or for patients with dyspnea who are taking weak opioids such as codeine, hydrocodone, or propoxyphene, consider switching to a strong oral opioid such as:

• **Oxycodone**—3-10 mg q 4 hours and prn

• **Morphine syrup**—3-10 mg q 4 hours and prn

• **Hydromorphone** (Dilaudid) **tablets**— 0.5-2 mg q 4 hours and prn

Severe Dyspnea Being Treated with Strong Opioids

With patients already taking strong opioids and with those with dyspnea and high levels of anxiety, try increasing the above doses by 50% every 4-12 hours until the patient experiences relief. An inpatient hospice/palliative care setting may be helpful and appropriate because close monitoring is essential and subcutaneous administration of escalating doses of opioids and midazolam (Versed) may be required. The entire interdisciplinary team should be involved in interventions for severe dyspnea.

Use of Oxygen

Opioids are the first-choice treatment agents for most nonspecific dyspnea associated with terminal illness. Because opioids are so effective, supplemental oxygen often is unnecessary in palliative care. When oxygen is required to help relieve severe dyspnea, nasal prongs may be all that is needed because opioids tend to reduce the patient's oxygen requirements. If possible, oxygen masks should be avoided because they are isolating and can be frightening.

Use of Naloxone (Narcan)

Ordering naloxone (Narcan) just because a terminally patient who is taking opioids is breathing less than 12-20 times a minute can be *extremely harmful.* Many terminally ill patients experience respirations of 6-12 per minute when asleep or awake. When terminally ill patients who have been on stable doses of opioids for several days develop decreased or erratic respirations in conjunction with weakness, decreased alertness, and cool extremities, the normal dying process has begun. The appropriate action is to talk with the patient's family about the dying process, *not* to give an order for naloxone. For more information, see the section, *Dispel Misconceptions about Morphine,* in *UNIPAC Three: Assessment and Treatment of Pain in the Terminally Ill.*

Opioids are not the cause of respiratory distress in patients who also are experiencing tachypnea and anxiety. As long as the patient is arousable, naloxone should not be administered. Naloxone should be reserved for rare cases such as accidental overdose and *should not* be administered in a way that completely reverses the effects of opioids in dying patients; such action can result in the return of extreme pain and precipitate a withdrawal crisis. Instead, for accidental overdoses, dilute 1 amp (0.4 mg) in 10 ml of saline and give 1 ml of this diluted mixture (0.04 mg) IV every 5 minutes until **partial** reversal occurs. This process may have to be repeated because naloxone has a shorter half-life than most opioids.

Continual Reassessment

Reevaluate continually to determine the need for different approaches to treatment such as the following:

- A caring listener for dyspnea complicated by isolation
- Benzodiazepines for dyspnea complicated by severe anxiety
- Steroids for dyspnea related to bronchospasm or suspected lymphangetic pulmonary spread of the cancer
- Thoracentesis for dyspnea complicated by a pleural effusion

Terminal Sedation

In most cases dyspnea can be adequately controlled with the following:
- Careful evaluation
- Specific treatment
- The general measures and use of opioids as outlined in this UNIPAC

However, in some cases, it may be necessary to administer high doses of parenteral opioids. Because dyspnea, like pain, directly antagonizes the sedative and respiratory depressant effects of opioids, patients with severe dyspnea can remain quite alert and breathe normally despite the use of high doses of opioids.

When patients are dying of respiratory failure, they frequently experience high levels of anxiety and restlessness, both of which are very distressing not only for the patient but also for family members, who are already experiencing high levels of stress. In such cases, the entire hospice/palliative care team must be involved in caring for both the patient **and** members of the family.

In some cases, when the symptoms of dyspnea are very severe, sedating the patient may be the most humane and appropriate action. The intent of the therapy always should be to relieve the patient's distress, even if unavoidable effects include loss of consciousness or possible shortening of the patient's life. Consider the following:

- Short-acting benzodiazepines are usually the easiest to titrate. Doses of lorazepam by mouth or sublingually or midazolam (Versed) subcutaneously can be started at low doses (0.25 mg per hour) but should be rapidly increased to reach the desired effect. Sometimes, as much as 2-3 mg per hour of subcutaneous midazolam (Versed) is required.[24] Midazolam (Versed) can be mixed with morphine or hydromorphone (Dilaudid) for subcutaneous infusion.

- Alternatives include chlorpromazine (Thorazine) 50-100 mg orally or by suppository every 2-8 hours or phenobarbital 60-130 mg orally or by subcutaneous bolus every hour as needed.

Clinical Situation Illustrating the Assessment and Treatment of Dyspnea

Clinical Situation: John and Alice O.

John is a 46-year-old male with a 30-year history of heavy smoking who was diagnosed 12 months ago with adenocarcinoma of the right lung. He is an insurance agent who lives with his wife and two children in a new, very attractive, four-bedroom house in the suburbs. John has been struggling to go to work every day despite radiation treatments and has refused chemotherapy.

When the physician first visits, John is experiencing shortness of breath when he walks across the room. He is using an albuterol inhaler 2 puffs three times a day, and taking theophylline slow-release 300 mg twice a day.

Question One

Which one of the following is the most appropriate first course of action?

[A] Prescribe oxygen 2 liters per minute by nasal prongs.

[B] Increase the theophylline to three times per day.

[C] Order a chest x-ray and arterial blood gases.

[D] Complete a thorough history and physical at the bedside.

Correct Response and Analysis

The correct answer is D. More information is needed before any decisions are made about medication orders or tests. The simple maneuver of completing a history and physical will cause the least amount of discomfort, risk, and expense, and is much more likely to provide productive information about which therapeutics to use. Oxygen may be helpful for dyspnea, but attachment to an oxygen concentrator limits mobility and John is still trying to get to work. If John is not wheezing, increasing his theophylline may only increase any agitation and tremulousness he may be experiencing without relieving his shortness of breath.

The Case Continues

Further discussion reveals John is using his albuterol inhaler approximately every hour during the day and is so tremulous and anxious he gets very little sleep at night. He is having moderate discomfort in his chest that he treats with acetaminophen and aspirin with only slight relief, but he refuses to take medications that might cause drowsiness because he wants to drive himself to work. An attempt at thoracentesis was made two weeks ago, but it was very painful and did not relieve John's dyspnea.

John is extremely angry at his employer, who has threatened to fire him because of his decreased work performance. John fears the likely cancellation of his health benefits and the loss of his home because, despite his career as an insurance agent, he had never purchased life insurance. He feels very guilty about the lack of insurance and the probability of his family having to leave their home as soon as his earnings stop. John's family is extremely stressed by his steady deterioration and increasing anger, which is often displaced on Alice and the children.

A physical examination reveals an angry, tremulous man who seems alert and clear-headed but appears older than his stated age. His vital signs are blood pressure 110/60, pulse 120, and respirations 30 times per minute. He has decreased breath sounds and scattered ronchi in both lung fields with absent breath sounds and dullness to percussion in the right lower lung field. His abdomen is soft with tenderness in the epigastric area but no palpable mass. His extremities show some muscle wasting and clubbing of his fingertips but no cyanosis or edema.

Question Two

At this point, effective interventions for John's shortness of breath include:

[A] Decrease the albuterol to 2 puffs tid and add prednisone 10 mg bid to help with bronchospasm.

[B] Involve a social worker and chaplain to address the family's financial problems and anguish about the future.

[C] Involve the hospice nurse to help John set reasonable limits on his activities to avoid exhaustion (use a wheelchair to conserve energy, allow family members to assist with family chores, allow someone to drive him to work, etc.).

[D] All of the above

Correct Response and Analysis

The correct response is D. Because the causes of dyspnea are multi-dimensional, treatment must address the physical, psychological, social, and spiritual components of shortness of breath.

The Case Continues

John's distress gradually improves as the above interventions are implemented. Several days later, lorazepam 1 mg at bedtime is added and John begins to sleep well. His family begins to cope much better. With help from the social worker, John is able to negotiate a "when-needed" unpaid 6-month leave of absence with his employer that allows him to retain his health insurance. Two weeks later, John experiences increasing shortness of breath on exertion and during the night. He is unable to return to work. John is not febrile or coughing up any sputum. The nurse listens to his chest and reports no major changes in his pulmonary exam.

Question Three

At this time the most appropriate intervention is:

[A] Order a CBC and type and cross-match for a possible blood transfusion.

[B] Order oxygen 2 liters by nasal prongs prn and acetaminophen with codeine (Tylenol #3) 1 tablet every 4-6 hours.

[C] Order a chest x-ray upright and supine to evaluate for possible effusions and need for thoracentesis.

[D] Order prednisone 40 mg bid to help with bronchospasm.

Correct Response and Analysis

The correct answer is B. Pneumonia seems unlikely in this situation, and after his bad experience with thoracentesis John is unlikely to accept another attempt. Ordering oxygen and acetaminophen with codeine is much less invasive and more likely to relieve the shortness of breath and discomfort related to John's lung cancer. It is important to warn John and his family about the possibility of codeine-induced nausea and to prescribe a laxative to prevent constipation caused by opioid therapy. For more information on the treatment of constipation, see *UNIPAC Three: Assessment and Treatment of Pain in the Terminally Ill*.

The Case Continues

John is much more comfortable at rest, but his acetaminophen with codeine (Tylenol #3) requirement increases to 2 tablets every 4 hours. Constipation is prevented with senna tablets. During the next visit, John is drowsy but breathing 40 times a minute with very few lung sounds in either base. He sleeps off and on throughout the day and night. He has 2-plus edema in his lower extremities, and the skin on his buttocks is reddened because he is comfortable only in an upright position. John's family is very distressed by his intermittent periods of severe dyspnea.

Question Four

At this time the most appropriate intervention is to:

[A] Order transdermal fentanyl (Duragesic patch) 25 mcg per hour.

[B] Order slow-release morphine (MS Contin or Oramorph SR) 30 mg bid.

[C] Order oxycodone with acetaminophen (Percocet) 1 tablet every 4 hours with an additional tablet in between as needed to relieve dyspnea.

[D] Order a morphine PCA pump at 1 mg per hour with a 1 mg booster dose as needed to relieve dyspnea.

Correct Response and Analysis

The correct response is C. Oxycodone with acetaminophen (Percocet) is likely to relieve shortness of breath and, unlike transdermal fentanyl or slow-release morphine, allows for careful dose titration and booster doses if needed. The large increase in opioid dosing from 2 tablets of acetaminophen with codeine (Tylenol #3) every 4 hours to 30 mg slow-release morphine or morphine 1 mg per hour by infusion pump is likely to result in oversedation. Transdermal fentanyl

(Duragesic patch) is not the preferred route because of highly variable absorption and the inability to rapidly titrate doses.

NOTE—See "Oral Morphine Equivalents" in *UNIPAC Three: Assessment and Treatment of Pain in the Terminally Ill.*

As John's shortness of breath is relieved, he may be willing to try other positions in bed to preserve the skin on his buttocks. Careful turning and special attention from the nursing staff will help prevent decubiti, as will a special mattress if the need arises.

The Case Concludes

John's shortness of breath is relieved by the oxycodone with acetaminophen (Percocet). During the next 2 weeks his opioid requirement gradually increases to 2 oxycodone with acetaminophen (Percocet) tablets every 4 hours with an additional booster dose as needed. Eventually, John is switched to oral and then to sublingual morphine 10-20 mg every 4 hours, which effectively controls his shortness of breath until he dies peacefully at home 3 weeks later. Alice is grateful for interventions provided by the hospice and the physician.

Nausea, Vomiting, and Bowel Obstruction

- Introduction to Nausea and Vomiting
- Pathophysiology of Vomiting
- Assessment and Treatment of Nausea and Vomiting
  - Principles of Treatment for Nausea
  - General Treatment Measures for Nausea
  - Specific Treatment Measures for Nausea
  - Persistent Nausea
  - Alternative Routes of Medication Delivery
    - SC Bolus Doses or Infusions
    - Rectal Suppositories
    - Other Suggestions
- Introduction to Bowel Obstruction
  - Symptoms of Bowel Obstruction
  - Surgical Treatment of Bowel Obstruction
  - Pharmacological Treatment of Bowel Obstruction
- Clinical Situation Illustrating the Assessment and Treatment of Nausea and Vomiting

Introduction to Nausea and Vomiting

In the terminally ill population, nausea and vomiting are symptoms that result from a variety of different causes, including the direct and indirect effects of several types of cancer. Nausea is more common than vomiting. In one series, 50% to 60% of terminally ill cancer patients experienced nausea compared with 30% of patients who experienced vomiting.[25] Both symptoms were most common among patients with stomach and breast cancers.

Nausea and vomiting are demoralizing complaints that can be controlled in more than 90% of terminally patients using the management techniques recommended in this module.[26]

Even the nausea associated with a complete bowel obstruction often can be palliated successfully without resorting to IVs or nasogastric tubes.[27, 28]

Pathophysiology of Vomiting

The pathophysiology of vomiting is better understood than that of many other symptoms. A section of the midbrain, referred to as the vomiting center, coordinates the vomiting reflex and receives input from the following sources:

- Cerebral cortex
- Inner ear (vestibular apparatus)
- Chemoreceptor trigger zone
- Gastrointestinal tract

Table 6

Pathophysiology of Vomiting

Intracranial pressure, Anxiety and memories	→ Cerebral Cortex	
Motion sickness, Vestibular disease	→ Vestibular Apparatus	→ Vomiting Center → Emesis
Uremia, Hypercalcemia drugs	→ Chemoreceptor Trigger Zone (floor of fourth ventricle)	
Gastric irritation, Intestinal distension, Gag reflex	→ Gastrointestinal tract	

Assessment and Treatment of Nausea and Vomiting

Because many factors contribute to nausea and vomiting, it is important to perform a careful history and physical to identify the specific contributing physical and psychosocial factors of each patient's case. The history and physical exam should focus on the identification of specific causes of nausea and vomiting (and other symptoms) so each problem can be individually treated.

During the history, special care should be taken to identify the relationship of symptoms to specific foods, drugs, movements, situations, odors, emotions, and thoughts. The possible concurrent presence of pain, dysphagia, and constipation should be considered and treated as needed. The physical exam should include an assessment of oral, abdominal, rectal, and neurological problems. In some cases, laboratory tests may be appropriate to assess the patient's serum levels of blood urea nitrogen, serum calcium, serum sodium, digoxin, or theophylline.

Principles of Treatment for Nausea

- When choosing a treatment, consider the etiology. See Table 7.

- Conditioned responses develop quickly so treatment should be prompt, prophylactic when possible, and tapered cautiously. When starting opioids, consider the prophylactic use of antiemetics for a few days. If nausea is recurrent, use regularly scheduled doses to prevent recurrence.

- Involve members of the interdisciplinary team to address the multiple physical, psychological, social, and spiritual problems that cause and exacerbate nausea and vomiting.

General Treatment Measures for Nausea

Encourage caregivers to:

- Provide small, frequent meals consisting of foods chosen by the patient.

- Provide liquids frequently.

- Provide a quiet, relaxing, pleasant atmosphere.

- Provide companionship for meals.

- Teach the patient relaxation techniques.

Encourage the patient to:
- Get enough rest.
- Avoid disagreeable foods and odors.
- Avoid fatty and fried foods.
- Try an alcoholic beverage before meals.
- Take most medications after eating (except antiemetics).

Specific Treatment Measures for Nausea

Specific measures for the treatment of nausea are included in Table 7.

Persistent Nausea

If nausea persists despite the use of the medications listed in Table 7, reevaluation is necessary. Reassess for specific causes and remedies such as the following:

- **Bowel obstruction**—see next section
- **Gastric compression from massive hepatomegaly**—consider higher dose PO or SC metoclopramide (Reglan) or cisapride (Propulsid)
- **Renal failure**—consider stent or SC antiemetic
- **Theophylline or digoxin toxicity**—reduce dose
- **Brain metastases**—consider high dose dexamethasone PO or SC

If no treatable cause can be found, a combination of antiemetics may be required.

Start with:
- Haloperidol 1 mg (by mouth if possible) bid to tid and push the dose to 10-15 mg per day if necessary

If needed, add:
- An antihistamine such as hydroxyzine 100-200 mg per day *and/or*
- Metoclopramide (Reglan) 40-80 mg per day

Table 7

Specific Measures for the Treatment of Nausea	
Specific Cause	**Possible Remedy**
Cortical	
• Tumor in CNS or meninges (look for neurologic signs or mental status problems)	• Dexamethasone (consider radiation therapy)
• Increased intracranial pressure (look for projectile vomiting, headache)	• Dexamethasone
• Anxiety and other conditioned responses	• Counseling, tranquilizers
• Uncontrolled pain	• Opioids, other pain medications
Vestibular/ Middle Ear	
• Vestibular disease (look for vertigo or vomiting after head motion)	• Meclizine and/or ENT consult
• Middle ear infections (look for ear pain or bulging tympanic membrane)	• Antibiotic and/or decongestant
• Motion sickness (travel-related nausea)	• Transderm Scop, meclizine
Chemoreceptor Trigger Zone	
The most common causes of nausea are mediated by this area in the brain, which senses changes in the blood.	
• Drugs, e.g., opioids, digoxin, chemotherapy, carbamazepine, antibiotics, theophylline	• Decrease drug dose or discontinue drug if possible
• Metabolic, e.g. renal or liver failure or tumor products	• Haloperidol PO or SC or ondansetron (Zofran) PO or SC
• Hyponatremia	• Salt tablets, demeclocycline
• Hypercalcemia	• Diphosphonate or other therapy

Table 7 (continued from page 43)

Specific Cause	Possible Remedy
Gastrointestinal Tract	
• Irritation by drugs, (e.g., NSAIDs, iron, alcohol, antibiotics)	• Stop drug if possible, add H_2 blocker or misoprostol
• Tumor infiltration, radiation therapy to the GI tract, or infection (e.g., candida esophagitis, colitis)	• Haloperidol SC, possibly with hydroxyzine SC or Transderm Scop
• Distention from constipation or impaction	• Laxative, manual disimpaction
• Obstruction by tumor or poor motility	• Metoclopramide (Reglan)
• Tube feedings	• Reduce feeding volume
• Gag reflex from feeding tube	• Remove it
• Nasopharyngeal bleeding	• Packing, vitamin K, sedation
• Thick secretions (cough-induced vomiting)	• Nebulized saline if good cough reflex, anticholinergic if poor cough reflex

Alternative Routes of Medication Delivery

SC Bolus Doses or Infusions

When patients cannot swallow or retain tablets, consider using subcutaneous bolus doses or infusions. Most families can be taught to give injections of the above medications into an injection site on a SC butterfly needle. The volume of drug given should be kept below 1.5 ml/injection to avoid discomfort. Change the injection site every 2-7 days. Alternatively, use a simple pump to deliver an infusion of medications subcutaneously.

- Combine the antiemetics (see Table 8) with the opioid the patient is taking, usually morphine or hydromorphone (Dilaudid).

- Give by continuous subcutaneous infusion through a 25-gauge butterfly needle, usually 1 ml every 2-6 hours. Higher volumes may require a continuous infusion.

- If haloperidol is given, use D5W as the diluent and keep the concentration of haloperidol below 1.5 mg per ml to avoid precipitation of haloperidol crystals.[29]
- The needle must be moved to a new location when the skin begins to get tender or inflamed, usually every 2-7 days.

Rectal Suppositories

- The same antiemetic agents may be delivered using custom-made rectal suppositories.
- Thorazine suppositories 25-100 mg every 4-8 hours can be effective and sedating.

Other Suggestions

- When treating severe persistent nausea with multiple causes, add dexamethasone either by mouth or by a separate SC injection site.
- Try the following medications, which are very expensive but may produce dramatically effective results when given orally (if tolerated) or by SC infusion:
  - Methotrimeprazine (Levoprome)[30] 50-300 mg/d
  - Ondansetron (Zofran)[31] 1 mg/hr
- Reassess continually for new complications.

Involve all members of the interdisciplinary team to help treat the social, psychological, and spiritual aspects of nausea and vomiting.

Table 8

Suggested Antiemetics for Parenteral Use

Agent	Compatible with SC tissues?	Compatible with Morphine or Dilaudid?[29]
Haloperidol (Haldol)	Yes	In 5% dextrose only
Metoclopramide (Reglan)	Yes	Yes
Hydroxyzine (Vistaril)	Yes	Yes
Methotrimeprazine	Yes (may require frequent new SC sites)	Yes
Dexamethasone	Yes	Only in small amounts
Chlorpromazine	No	Yes
Promethazine	No	Yes

Introduction to Bowel Obstruction

The incidence of bowel obstruction ranges from 5.5% to 42% in patients with ovarian cancer and from 10% to 28.4% in patients with colorectal malignancies.[28] Gastrointestinal obstruction occurs in approximately 3% of patients with advanced cancer who are receiving hospice care.[27] Bowel obstructions are caused by intestinal muscle paralysis (paralytic ileus) or occlusion of the lumen (mechanical ileus) or both. An obstruction can be partial, complete, single, or multiple, and can result from benign causes, inflammatory bowel disease, or malignancy.[28]

Symptoms of Bowel Obstruction

Although bowel obstructions can occur at any time during a cancer patient's clinical history, they tend to develop more often and more quickly during the advanced stage of illness.[32] However, when bowel obstruction occurs in terminal cancer patients, onset is rarely an acute event. The following three symptoms are almost always present:

- Intestinal colic (cramping, intermittent pain)
- Abdominal pain due to distention, hepatomegaly, or tumor masses
- Nausea and/or vomiting that may be intermittent or continuous

Other symptoms include abdominal distention, visible peristalsis, intermittent borborygmi (high-pitched, loud, bowel sounds), and anorexia. Although complete bowel obstruction presents with constipation for feces and flatus, overflow diarrhea may result from bacterial liquefaction of the fecal material blocked in the colon or rectum. Partial obstruction, as by a fecal impaction, is another common cause of diarrhea. Constipation and simple paralytic ileus should be ruled out, if possible, by abdominal x-rays or therapeutic trials of laxatives and enemas.[28]

Surgical Treatment of Bowel Obstruction

Even when patients are fit enough to undergo a colostomy or intestinal bypass, surgery might not be the best option because it may not successfully relieve problems associated with obstruction; a large percentage of patients experience further complications.[28] In one study, only 56% of patients survived 60 days after surgery, and 43% of the survivors continued to experience intermittent symptoms of both complete and incomplete intestinal obstruction until death occurred.[33]

Pharmacological Treatment of Bowel Obstruction

When terminally ill patients in the hospice/palliative care setting develop bowel obstructions, the therapeutic goal is to manage the symptoms and maximize quality of life. Diverting surgery should be considered but often will prove impractical due to the patient's weakened condition from advanced terminal illness and multiple sites of obstruction. Successful symptom control can be achieved using analgesic, anticholinergic, and antiemetic drugs without the use of decompression tubes, surgery, or intravenous fluids.[28]

When symptoms associated with bowel obstruction are treated, the following points should be considered:

- The route of drug administration must be personalized—medication dosages and combinations initially will require frequent readjustment.

- Vomiting may prohibit oral administration of drugs.

- Rectal and sublingual routes for some drugs are safe and effective for home settings. Sublingual route use may be limited by nausea, and use of the rectal route may be limited by patient modesty, the lack of availability of custom-made suppositories, overflow diarrhea, and the discomfort of rectally administering multiple drugs every 4 hours.

- Continuous subcutaneous infusion using a portable pump is recommended because it allows for parenteral administration of different combinations of drugs, causes minimal discomfort, and is easy to use in a home or inpatient setting.

- When central venous catheters are already in place, they may be used to administer drugs. Inserting new catheters is painful and unnecessary.

- A venting gastrostomy may be helpful for high-grade proximal obstructions, but nasogastric suction and intravenous fluids for symptom control are uncomfortable and rarely necessary or helpful for long-term use.

- When symptoms are controlled, quality of life improves, not only because symptom relief has been achieved but also because patients may be able to drink fluids and eat small amounts of favorite foods.

- Remember the therapeutic goal—no pain, no cramps, minimal nausea, and no more than one emesis per day. Consider the treatments in Table 9.

Nausea, Vomiting, and Bowel Obstruction

Table 9

Pharmacological Treatment of Pain, Nausea, and Constipation Associated with Bowel Obstruction

Drug	Dose	Comment
Pain		
Morphine or hydromorphone	Titrate to relief PO, SL, SC, or IV (Remember, morphine SC dose = 1/3 PO dose and hydromorphone SC dose = 1/5 PO dose)	For cramping pain (colic), may need high dosage or addition of glycopyrrolate (Robinul) 0.4-1.0 mg/d SC or hyoscyamine (Levsin SL) 0.125 mg SL q 4-8 hours. If pain unrelieved, consider celiac plexus block.
Nausea		
Haloperidol (Haldol)	5-15 mg/d SC,PO, or IV	Mix in 5% dextrose for SC infusion.
Metoclopramide (Reglan)	60-240 mg/d SC, PO, or IV	May cause colic unless combined with a high dose opioid.
Hydroxyzine (Vistaril)	100-200 mg/d SC, PO, or IV	Add to haloperidol if necessary.
Chlorpromazine (Thorazine)	25-100 mg/tid PO, PR, or IV	Suppositories useful if SC infusion of above agents is unavailable. Sedating.
Methotrimeprazine (Levoprome)	50-300 mg/d SC or IV	Expensive, analgesic, sedating, but very effective. May need daily change of SC site.
Persistent Vomiting of Secretions (despite above measures)		
Octreotide (Sandostatin)	0.1-0.6 mg/d by SC infusion	Expensive, reduces GI secretions.[34]
Constipation (in subtotal obstruction)		
Docusate	100 mg PO bid-q 4 hours	Stimulant laxative like senna or bisacodyl, may cause colic.
Dexamethasone	4 mg PO or SC bid-qid	May relieve obstruction, but discontinue if ineffective after 5 days.

Clinical Situation Illustrating the Assessment and Treatment of Nausea and Vomiting

Clinical Situation: Selena and Mariana Q.

Selena is a 58-year-old widow with advanced breast cancer who is barely able to move from her bed to the bedside commode. She has undergone several rounds of chemotherapy and radiation to her chest wall, right arm, and left hip. Selena is moderately obese with a very edematous right arm. During the hospice team's first visit, her principal complaints are nausea and pain in her right arm. The nausea is so severe that Selena's oral intake has been limited to clear liquids. For the past 2 days she has been unable to tolerate her medicines, which has resulted in a substantial increase in her pain. Selena is being cared for by her daughter, Mariana.

Selena's medications are piroxicam (Feldene) 20 mg daily, slow-release morphine (MS Contin) 30 mg bid, and theophylline slow-release (Theo-Dur) 300 mg bid.

Question One

At this point, which one of the following is the most appropriate intervention?

[A] Order prochlorperazine (Compazine) 5 mg q 4 hours as needed.

[B] Complete a more thorough history and physical.

[C] Order promethazine (Phenergan) suppositories 25 mg q 4 hours prn.

[D] Discontinue all PO medications and order morphine 2 mg per hour IV.

[E] None of the above

Correct Response and Analysis

The correct response is B. As always, more information is needed before any decisions are made about medication orders or tests. The simple maneuver of completing a history and physical will cause the least amount of discomfort, risk, and expense, and is much more likely to provide productive information about which therapeutic strategy to use.

The Case Continues

Further history reveals that Selena has been mildly nauseated for some time, but her nausea increased dramatically 2 days ago when her family physician changed her pain medication from acetaminophen 300 mg with codeine 30 mg (Tylenol #3) 1 tablet every 4 hours as needed to slow-release morphine 30 mg twice daily. Selena has been drowsy and nauseated ever since, and she has not had a bowel movement for 4 days. She says her abdomen feels as if it is distended and she feels nauseated all the time, in particular at meal time.

The piroxicam (Feldene) 20 mg Selena has been taking for 2 years was first prescribed for osteoarthritic pain but is now used to relieve pain related to her bone metastases. She has a history of mild bronchitis but experiences no shortness of breath at this time and has never been told she has asthma.

A physical exam reveals a blood pressure of 110/60 and a regular pulse of 100. Selena has a normal heart rate and rhythm and no murmurs. Her chest has scattered ronchi. She has obviously had a right-sided mastectomy and has skin changes on the right upper chest from radiation therapy. Her right arm is grossly swollen with lymphedema.

Selena's abdomen is distended but her obesity makes it difficult to tell if she has masses or ascites. Although she is experiencing generalized abdominal discomfort, she reports no specific area of abdominal pain. She has some increased tenderness in the suprapubic area and on further questioning reports she has to urinate every hour but can pass only small amounts of urine each time. A rectal exam reveals soft stool and mild tenderness in the rectal area. Her lower extremities show some muscle wasting and edema but no cyanosis.

During the exam Selena is alert and oriented and answers questions appropriately, but she seems miserable and depressed.

Question Two

To control Selena's nausea, which of the following are appropriate maneuvers?

[A] Discontinue the piroxicam (Feldene) 20 mg because of potential gastritis that may contribute to nausea.

[B] Discontinue the theophylline slow-release (Theo-Dur) 300 mg bid to avoid potential theophylline toxicity that may contribute to nausea, and substitute an albuterol inhaler.

[C] Discontinue the slow-release morphine 30 mg bid and substitute oxycodone 5 mg plus acetaminophen 325 mg (Percocet) every 4 hours because the rapid escalation in opioid dose may be contributing to her nausea and urinary retention.

[D] Add a laxative for constipation and an antacid for potential gastritis.

[E] All of the above

Correct Response and Analysis

The correct response is E. Discontinuing the medications Selena was taking and substituting more appropriate drugs will help improve her situation.

The Case Continues

The physician prescribes acetaminophen 325 mg with oxycodone 5 mg (Percocet) one tablet every 4 hours for Selena's discomfort, an albuterol inhaler as needed for her bronchitis, and an appropriate laxative and antacid. Three days later, the home care nurse reports that Selena is much improved; her pain and nausea are adequately controlled, her bowels and bladder are working better, and her spirits have improved dramatically.

Four weeks later, Selena's pain increases. When an increase in the dose of pain medication from 1 tablet of acetaminophen 325 mg with oxycodone 5 mg (Percocet) every 4 hours to 2 tablets every 4 hours is no longer effective, the physician prescribes slow-release morphine 30 mg every 12 hours with metoclopramide (Reglan) 10 mg tid for 3 days to prevent nausea. After the metoclopramide is discontinued, Selena is able to continue the oral morphine without experiencing nausea.

Two weeks later, Mariana reports that Selena has been eating regularly, but now she is nauseated much of the day and is vomiting twice a day after she eats. She is barely able to tolerate her oral morphine and laxative, but she is having regular bowel movements.

The physician makes a home visit to reevaluate the situation and finds Selena is still able to give short, appropriate answers to simple questions but is much weaker than when last seen. She also is obviously in distress from her nausea and increased pain in her right arm.

The physical exam shows her condition is unchanged from before, except for increased weakness, decreased obesity, and a Stage I decubitus forming on her buttocks. Selena's abdomen is mildly tender, particularly in the right upper quadrant, where a tender, enlarged liver can now be felt. She has no epigastric tenderness and no signs of bladder distention in the suprapubic area. Bowel sounds are rare, and her rectum reveals only a small amount of soft stool.

Question Three

At this point, in addition to increasing Selena's slow-release morphine dose to 60 mg bid and caring for her decubitus, appropriate interventions to control nausea include which of the following:

[A] Order metoclopramide (Reglan) 10 mg before each meal and at bedtime.

[B] Order promethazine (Phenergan) 25 mg PO tid.

[C] Order haloperidol (Haldol) 1 mg bid for nausea.

[D] Any of the above

Correct Response and Analysis

The correct response is D. Any of the listed interventions is likely to improve Selena's situation because each of them helps relieve chemoreceptor trigger zone-induced nausea. The haloperidol is less sedating than the promethazine, and the metoclopramide improves gut motility.

The Case Continues

With medication to control nausea, Selena's nausea and vomiting decrease. She begins to drink liquids and eat small amounts of soft food, but she is drowsy and sleeps most of the time. She is often confused and sometimes hallucinates. Mariana is unhappy about her mother's deterioration and threatens to stop giving the medications unless something can be done to relieve her mother's symptoms with fewer sedating complications.

After a physical exam, the hospice nurse reports that Selena's condition is unchanged, except her mental state has deteriorated. **NOTE**—At this point, it can be difficult to determine whether mental changes are the result of reversible problems. The physician considers three possibilities: checking Selena's serum calcium and electrolytes, beginning an empiric trial of steroids for CNS mets, and prescribing antibiotics for possible infection.

Because the nurse examined Selena just a few days ago and found her to be extremely weak, with no evidence of these reversible problems, the physician decides that Selena's deterioration in mental status is most likely irreversible.

Question Four

Which of the following are appropriate maneuvers to improve Selena's mental status and control her nausea and pain?

[A] Transfer Selena to a hospice inpatient unit for further evaluation, initiation of a subcutaneous infusion, and family respite.

[B] At home, begin morphine 30-40 mg per day and metoclopramide (Reglan) 30 mg per day by continuous subcutaneous infusion. **NOTE**— Selena was on slow-release morphine 60 mg bid. To convert morphine from an oral to an injectable dose, calculate the patient's daily oral dose of morphine (in this case 120 mg) and divide by 3, which in this case equals 40 mg per day. For information on conversions, see *UNIPAC Three: Assessment and Treatment of Pain in the Terminally Ill*.

[C] Substitute hydromorphone (Dilaudid) 4 mg PO q 4 hours and metoclopramide (Reglan) 10 mg q 8 hours for the pain and nausea medications.

[D] Decrease the slow-release morphine dose to 30 mg q 8 hours, add naproxen (Naprosyn) 375 mg tid with misoprostol (Cytotec) 200 mcg tid to protect her stomach, and change the antiemetic to haloperidol (Haldol) 2 mg per day at bedtime.

[E] Any of the above

Correct Response and Analysis

The correct response is E. In most patient care situations, any of several appropriate management strategies is likely to improve the patient's situation. Each of the listed maneuvers is likely to improve Selena's mental status and control her pain and nausea because each either reduces the morphine dose, changes the medication delivery route, rotates to a different opioid, and uses a less-sedating antiemetic. If the physician strongly suspects a reversible cause, option A might be most appropriate.

The Case Concludes

The chosen intervention temporarily improves Selena's mental status and adequately controls her pain and nausea.

As Selena continues to weaken, it becomes clear she is dying. When she begins to experience difficulty swallowing, either the infusion is continued or the hospice nurse teaches Mariana to give the slow-release morphine rectally and to give haloperidol (Haldol) 1 mg tid subcutaneously using a butterfly needle in the subcutaneous tissues with an injection site. These maneuvers effectively control Selena's discomfort and nausea until she dies 1 week later. Mariana is grateful to the physician and the hospice team for their interventions and for listening to her concerns.

Delirium and Terminal Restlessness

- Introduction to Delirium and Terminal Restlessness
- Delirium
  - Assessment for Delirium
  - Treatment of Delirium
  - Treatment of Severe Agitated Delirium
- Restlessness
  - Assessment for Restlessness
  - Treatment of Restlessness
- Clinical Situation Illustrating the Assessment and Treatment of Delirium and Terminal Restlessness

Introduction to Delirium and Terminal Restlessness

Delirium and terminal restlessness or agitation are commonly experienced by terminally ill patients during the final stages of life. These symptoms are often extremely distressing for both patients and families. Although the presence of clear mentation distinguishes restlessness from delirium, the two symptoms often occur together.

Delirium

Assessment for Delirium

Up to 85% of terminally ill cancer patients experience delirium, a symptom that is distressing for both patients and family members, especially when it is accompanied by calling out, attempts to climb over bed rails, and obvious terror.

Delirium is characterized by the following DSM-IV criteria:[35]

- Clouding of consciousness or reduced ability to focus, sustain, or shift attention
- Perceptual disturbance, disorientation, or memory deficit that is not better accounted for by an established dementia
- Acute onset (hours to days) and a fluctuating course
- General evidence from the history and physical or laboratory findings of a medical condition related to the disturbance

Differentiating delirium from dementia can be difficult because they share clinical features such as disorientation and impaired thinking and judgment; however, the onset of delirium is an acute phenomenon, rather than a chronically progressive one, as with dementia. Remember that delirium may be superimposed on underlying dementia, particularly in elderly patients and those with AIDS.

A complete review of the patient's medications and physical condition is warranted. If possible and appropriate, consider reducing the patient's sedatives, treating hypercalcemia, or treating an infection. Some authors recommend a trial of rehydration by hypodermoclycis if the patient is dehydrated and confused.[36] Unfortunately, these efforts are unsuccessful most of the time. In one series, efforts to improve the cognitive function of patients with advanced cancer (by reducing or discontinuing a drug, managing electrolytes, or prescribing antibiotics or steroids) helped only 18% of patients.[37]

Table 10 lists the most common causes of delirium.

Table 10
Common Causes of Delirium

D	**Drugs,** especially psychotropics
E	**Electrolyte** or glucose abnormality
L	**Liver** failure
I	**Ischemia** or hypoxia
R	**Renal** failure
I	**Impaction** of stool
U	**Urinary** tract or other infection
M	**Metastases** to the brain

Treatment of Delirium

When strategies to reverse the delirium are unsuccessful or inappropriate, as is usually the case, a neuroleptic can help calm the patient and improve mentation. Consider:

- **Haloperidol** (Haldol)—1-2 mg PO or SC hourly as needed to calm a crisis, then q 6-12 hours PO or by infusion

If more sedation is needed or for AIDS dementia complex, consider:

- **Thioridazine** (Mellaril)—25-50 mg PO hourly until calm, then q 6-12 hours

OR

- **Chlorpromazine** (Thorazine)—25-50 mg PO, PR, or IV hourly until calm, then q 6-12 hours or by infusion

Treatment of Severe Agitated Delirium

For severe agitated delirium, consider the addition of benzodiazepines or a high dose of a sedating phenothiazine, even though they may cause more clouding of the sensorium. Try:

- **Lorazepam** (Ativan)—1-2 mg hourly, orally or sublingually
- **Midazolam** (Versed)—0.4-4 mg/hour continuous SC (a mean dose of 2.9 mg/hr [70 mg/day] was effective in 22 of 23 patients in one series)[38]
- **Chlorpromazine** (Thorazine)—100 mg every hour IV, PO, PR
- **Methotrimeprazine** (Levoprome)—20 mg IM or IV every hour can help with agitation, pain, and nausea in a crisis

Some patients are helped by a combination of:

- **Haloperidol** (Haldol)—5-20 mg/day and midazolam (Versed) 10-100 mg/day via continuous subcutaneous infusion

In rare cases, when none of the above methods works during the final hours of a patient's life, consider:

- **Phenobarbital**—130 mg SC hourly until calm and then by subcutaneous infusion (600-1200 mg/day)[39]

When all else fails, consider:

- **Thiopental**—(20-200 mg/hr) or methohexital sodium (Brevital Sodium) continuous IV infusion titrated to unconsciousness[40, 41]

NOTE—The use of profound sedation to control severe, agitated delirium and restlessness in terminally ill patients is based on informed consent and an acknowledgment of the ethical principle of "double effect."[41] For more information on the principle of double effect, please see *UNIPAC Six: Ethical and Legal Decision Making When Caring for the Terminally Ill.* The desired effects of controlling severe agitated delirium and restlessness with deep sedation are relief of the patient's distressing physical symptoms and decreased suffering. Undesired effects may include loss of the ability to relate to others, loss of consciousness, and possible shortening of life.

When invoking the principle of double effect, clinicians must clearly intend the relief of distressing symptoms as the desired outcome.[41] Without this understanding, the moral reservations of health professionals or family members may result in either undertreatment of symptoms with continued patient suffering or subsequent guilt with its attendant consequences.[41]

For more information on treating difficult symptoms during the final days and hours of a patient's life and related ethical and communication issues, please refer to the following UNIPACs:

- UNIPAC Two: Psychological, Spiritual, and Physiological Aspects of Dying and Bereavement
- UNIPAC Five: Caring for the Terminally Ill: Communication and the Interdisciplinary Team Approach
- UNIPAC Six: Ethical and Legal Decision Making When Caring for the Terminally Ill

Restlessness

Assessment of Restlessness

During the assessment process, a complete and diligent review of the patient's medications and physical condition is important because treatable causes of restlessness often are present.

Consider any changes in the patient's condition, including the following:

- Is pain a contributing factor? Is the patient now too weak to articulate the cause of distress or to swallow oral medications? Try an increase in the analgesic dose or an alternative route of opioid delivery.
- Has a sedating drug been added? Is it helping?
- Is low sodium or high calcium a factor?
- Is kidney or liver failure a factor?
- Do focal neurologic signs suggest a cerebral metastasis?
- Is a fecal impaction present? Try an enema and institute a bowel regimen.
- Is urinary retention present? No drug relieves the pain of a blocked Foley catheter!
- Are psychosocial factors contributing? Fear, financial concerns, unresolved relationship issues, and anxiety can cause severe restlessness.
- Are spiritual problems contributing? Guilt and existential anguish can cause restlessness. Is the patient too weak to articulate his/her suffering?

Treatment of Restlessness

The physical causes of restlessness such as those listed in the previous section should be treated first. The physician also should explore psychosocial and spiritual issues with the patient and coordinate intervention efforts with appropriate members of the interdisciplinary team, including counselors, social workers, and/or chaplains. When fears of being alone contribute to restlessness, the continued presence of calming family members, friends, or hospice volunteers can help alleviate the patient's distress. The patient may appreciate distraction activities such as soft music or the sound of a person's voice reading aloud.

Although an unfamiliar environment can intensify both restlessness and delirium, consider transferring the patient to a hospice/palliative care inpatient unit. A brief stay in the unit's homelike atmosphere can be an effective diagnostic and therapeutic maneuver, particularly when family stress may be exacerbating the patient's symptoms or when family members are feeling unable to cope with the patient's distressing behavior.

When no specific problem can be identified and treated and the patient continues to suffer from anxiety and restlessness, consider carefully titrated doses of:

- **Lorazepam** (Ativan)—0.5-2 mg q 4 hours prn PO or SL,

or

- **Midazolam** (Versed)—2-60 mg per day continuous SC

When the above measures fail to control severe anxiety and terminal restlessness, see the previous section, *Treatment for Severe Agitated Delirium.*

Clinical Situation Illustrating the Assessment of Delirium and Terminal Restlessness

Clinical Situation: Sidney and Madeline

Sidney is a 71-year-old male with lung cancer metastatic to his bones and chest wall. When Sidney was first admitted to the hospice service as a home care patient, his 70-year-old wife, Madeline, was distressed because Sidney was in pain and sleeping poorly. Sidney's physician had prescribed acetaminophen with codeine (Tylenol #3) on an as-needed basis, but the medication was not providing adequate pain relief, even though Sidney took it on a regular basis.

With the help of the entire interdisciplinary team, Sidney's condition is improving. The hospice physician has prescribed the following: oxycodone 5 mg (Roxicodone) one tablet every 4 hours, lorazepam 1 mg at bedtime for sleep, a laxative, and a hospital bed so Madeline can care for Sidney more easily. A hospice volunteer visits every afternoon so Madeline can rest or take a nap.

This regimen works well for 2 weeks, but Sidney's condition deteriorates and he begins to have more problems with daytime sleepiness and confusion. The lorazepam dose is reduced and the nurse encourages Sidney to stay awake as much as possible during the day so he can sleep at night, but Sidney is growing weaker and eating less. At 10 pm on Friday, the hospice on-call nurse receives a call from Madeline, who reports that Sidney is agitated, refusing to swallow his tablets, and calling out for help.

Question One

At this point, the most appropriate intervention is:

[A] Complete a thorough history and physical.

[B] Hospitalize Sidney in an inpatient psychiatric facility.

[C] Order chlorpromazine (Thorazine) 100 mg IM.

[D] Discontinue all medications.

[E] Tell Madeline the symptoms are normal and must be endured.

Correct Response and Analysis

The correct response is A. As always, more information is needed before any decisions are made about medication orders or tests. The simple maneuver of completing a history and physical will cause the least amount of discomfort, risk, and expense and is much more likely to provide productive information about which therapeutics to use.

The Case Continues

When the hospice on-call nurse arrives, she discovers that Sidney has been refusing to take his prescribed oxycodone (Roxicodone) tablets on a regular schedule for the past 2 days, he has not had a bowel movement for 3 days, and he has been somewhat agitated since morning. Due to Sidney's agitation and hallucinations, Madeline has given him an extra lorazepam tablet twice that day.

Because Sidney is suspicious and uncooperative, the physical exam is very difficult to perform, but the nurse is able to determine that Sidney's pulse is 120, his skin is somewhat dry, he has decreased breath sounds on both sides of his chest, his abdomen is mildly distended, and he has a prominent mass in the suprapubic area. His extremities show muscle wasting and edema. Sidney will not allow the nurse to check his blood pressure.

Question Two

Likely causes of Sidney's agitation include which of the following:

[A] Fecal impaction

[B] Oxycodone (Roxicodone) overdose

[C] Urinary retention

[D] Early delirium

[E] Sedative overdose

Correct Response and Analysis

The correct responses are A, C, D, and E. Sidney is delirious. Both fecal impaction and urinary retention can cause agitation. The lorazepam, in particular the extra dose Sidney received, may be contributing. An oxycodone (Roxicodone) overdose is unlikely because Sidney's maintenance dose is small and he has not been taking it regularly for several days. Brain metastases are an additional possibility, particularly with lung cancer, but are unlikely because there are no focal neurologic signs or signs of increased intracranial pressure such as headaches or nausea. Electrolyte abnormalities or an infection also are possible, but obvious problems should be addressed first.

The Case Continues

The nurse calls the hospice physician, who orders chlorpromazine (Thorazine) 25 mg IM and oxycodone (Roxicodone), which the nurse crushes and convinces Sidney to eat in some pudding. Within 30 minutes Sidney is calm enough for the nurse to insert a Dulcolax suppository and help him to the bathroom, where he is able to expel a fecal impaction and partially empty his full bladder. A Foley catheter is inserted and Sidney drifts off to sleep.

NOTE—In this situation the use of chlorpromazine (Thorazine) can calm the patient enough to initiate other needed interventions, for example, treating the constipation and urinary retention, even though it is sedating and has anticholinergic side effects.

The next morning, Sidney is drowsy but less distressed. The hospice physician changes Sidney's medication to oral morphine 5 mg every 4 hours because it is easier to swallow. The physician also discontinues the lorazepam and starts thioridazine (Mellaril) 25 mg at bedtime as needed for sleep, and changes the laxative to bisacodyl tablets 5 mg twice a day because the tablets are easier to swallow. Biscodyl suppositories are ordered on an as-needed basis if Sidney does not have a bowel movement for 2 days.

These medications are much easier for Sidney to take and, with Madeline's help, Sidney remains comfortable for the next 3 days, despite his deteriorating strength and mental clarity. During this time the hospice social worker and chaplain visit with Sidney and Madeline to provide support and to gently inquire about the presence of psychosocial and/or spiritual issues that might be contributing to Sidney's agitation. Sidney and Madeline communicate openly about their concerns, but no serious complicating issues are uncovered.

On Tuesday (4 days after the crisis) the hospice nurse finds Sidney in bed and drowsy, but he can be aroused and seems comfortable as he drifts back to sleep. He has eaten very little for the past 2 days. In an attempt to improve Sidney's mental clarity, the nurse and physician confer with Madeline and together they decide to decrease the oral morphine to 3 mg every 4 hours. Madeline is reminded that the thioridazine (Mellaril) should be used only if needed for restlessness.

The next day Madeline reports that Sidney is less drowsy but he is complaining of increased chest wall pain. The physician suggests adding naproxen, but the nurse is concerned about Sidney's ability to swallow an additional medication. Madeline is becoming worried about her continued ability to care for Sidney at night because Sidney's agitation seems to be increasing. The physician and nurse discuss inpatient care, but Madeline decides she wants to continue to care for Sidney at home with the help of a hospice home health aide. Indomethacin (Indocin) suppositories 50 mg every 8 hours are prescribed for the chest wall pain.

At 11 pm on Thursday, the on-call nurse receives a desperate call from Madeline, who reports that her daughter has arrived from out of town and that they are extremely upset about Sidney's worsening agitation. Sidney is trying to climb over the bed rails, is reaching for spiders and snakes he sees in his bed, and is calling out for help. He is unwilling to swallow the thioridazine (Mellaril), and an additional dose of morphine does not improve the situation. The hospice nurse visits and finds Sidney's physical condition the same as before, except his Foley catheter is in place and working. Madeline reports that Sidney had a bowel movement earlier in the day.

Question Three

At this point, which of the following are appropriate interventions?

[A] Order sublingual morphine and chlorpromazine (Thorazine) suppositories 50 mg every 6 hours for restlessness.

[B] Order continuous SC morphine at 10 mg per day with haloperidol (Haldol) 5 mg per day and midazolam (Versed) 5 mg per day.

[C] Order lorazepam 1 mg by mouth as needed.

[D] Order restraints for his chest and hands.

[E] Increase involvement of the entire interdisciplinary team for family support.

Correct Response and Analysis

Correct responses are A or B, and E. Either the chlorpromazine (Thorazine) suppositories with sublingual morphine or the continuous subcutaneous mixture of morphine, haloperidol (Haldol), and midazolam (Versed) are likely to improve Sidney's condition. In either case, increased involvement of the entire interdisciplinary team is needed to help Sidney and his family cope with his increasing restlessness, delirium, and approaching death. C is incorrect because lorezapam has been tried already, and, in Sidney's case, it worsened the delirium. D is incorrect because restraints are not the most humane way of managing restlessness and delirium in any patient, particularly for one who is terminally ill.

The Case Concludes

Sidney refuses the suppositories. A subcutaneous line is started, but Sidney soon rips it out, even though he has received several boosts of the morphine, haloperidol (Haldol), and midazolam (Versed) mixture. The nurse again offers inpatient care, but Madeline refuses, despite her daughter's concern about their ability to manage Sidney at home.

Although somewhat uncomfortable in this situation, the physician orders haloperidol (Haldol) 5 mg IM or SC every 10 minutes until Sidney is calm. After the nurse gives three doses, Sidney is less agitated but still reaches out occasionally. The continuous subcutaneous infusion is restarted, this time above Sidney's shoulder blade, where he is less likely to disturb it, and the mixture is increased to morphine 10 mg, haloperidol (Haldol) 15 mg, and midazolam (Versed) 20 mg per 24 hours. Because the continuous infusion is delivered via a 25-gauge butterfly, it is unlikely to cause problems even if Sidney lies down on it.

Sidney is now calmer and allows the nurse to insert three of the chlorpromazine (Thorazine) 25 mg suppositories. After Sidney drifts off to sleep, the nurse shows the family how to give boosts of the subcutaneous infusion in the event Sidney awakens and is restless.

The next morning Sidney is very drowsy, but Madeline and her daughter are able to arouse him to give him sips of water. Sidney now requires 50 mg of chlorpromazine (Thorazine) bid by rectum. In the evening his restlessness and delirium increase, so his subcutaneous infusion medication doses are increased by 50% to morphine 15 mg, haloperidol (Haldol) 22 mg, and midazolam (Versed) 30 mg. These measures allow Sidney to remain at home as he wishes, and he dies comfortably the next day. Madeline and her daughter are very grateful to the physician and the entire hospice team for their interventions.

NOTE—Although research is limited, it is not uncommon for terminally ill patients to experience difficulties with restlessness or delirium during the active phase of dying that require frequent adjustments in medications, dosages, and routes of delivery. With diligent effort and use of methods such as those described in this clinical situation, most restlessness can be controlled. To control symptoms in patients with extremely severe agitation, medication doses may need to be increased substantially from "standard" doses and may need to be even higher than those described in this clinical situation.

Because the symptoms of agitated terminal restlessness are so distressing for the patient and family, it is important to treat symptoms aggressively. When state laws permit, hospice on-call nurses can be equipped with injectable or rectal sedatives so treatment of severe symptoms can begin without unnecessary delay. In addition, the entire interdisciplinary team should be involved in such cases and should make frequent home visits to provide support for the family.

Pretest Correct Responses

1. **False.** In most cases, treating reversible physical causes of anorexia such as constipation or oral candidiasis is more likely to be effective. Patient and family guilt about lack of appetite must also be addressed. These measures usually suffice. (See Table 3 and pages 12-13)

2. **False.** Tubes and diverting surgery usually are unnecessary for terminally ill patients. In most cases successful symptom control can be achieved using analgesics, anticholinergics, and antiemetic drugs given by SC infusion without the use of decompression tubes, surgery, or intravenous fluids. (See page 47)

3. **True.** Acute onset (hours to days) and a fluctuating course help distinguish delirium from dementia. (See page 56)

4. **True.** Carefully titrated opioids are effective treatments for dyspnea because they suppress respiratory awareness, decrease breathlessness, and increase exercise tolerance. (See page 29)

5. **True.** Some antiemitics such as haloperidol (Haldol), metoclopramide (Reglan), and hydroxyzine (Vistoril) can be combined with an opioid in a subcutaneous infusion. (See page 45)

6. **True.** When reassessment reveals no treatable causes of nausea, parenteral antiemetics may be used to control severe persistent nausea. (See page 42)

7. **True.** Although parenteral hydration by hypodermoclysis may have a role in the treatment of intractable thirst or delirium in some patients, in most cases artificial nutrition or hydration in the final days of life will result in more burden than benefit due to increased secretions, ascites, or effusions. (See pages 13 and 56)

8. **True.** These are common causes of delirium, as are hepatic or renal failure, stool impaction, and brain metastases. (See page 57)

9. **True.** Like pain and many other distressing symptoms such as nausea and restlessness, dyspnea is a complicated symptom with multiple physical, emotional, and spiritual components. (See page 26)

10. **True.** When no reversible etiology can be identified or when other treatments do not completely alleviate symptoms, opioids are first-choice agents for treating nonspecific dyspnea associated with terminal illness because they are so effective. (See page 29)

Pretest Correct Responses

11. **False.** A thorough assessment and treatment of reversible physical conditions are appropriate first steps when treating anorexia. (See page 10)

12. **False.** Reversible causes of dry mouth such as anticholinergic drugs and severe anxiety should be treated first. Inexpensive interventions also include a room humidifier or frequent drips of water from a syringe or foam toothbrush. (See Table 4 on page 16)

13. **False.** Carefully titrated doses of opioids are unlikely to result in clinically significant respiratory depression; many terminally ill patients breath less than 12 times per minute when asleep or awake. (See page 30)

14. **True.** Mild dyspnea often responds to treatment with a weak opioid such as hydrocodone. (See page 29)

15. **True.** Metoclopramide (Reglan) is compatible with subcutaneous tissues and can be combined with hydromorphone (Dilaudid) or morphine for the effective treatment of persistent nausea. (See page 45)

16. **False.** Tranquilizers may be an effective treatment for nausea mediated by the cerebral cortex but are unlikely to be effective in nausea mediated by the vestibular zone; other treatments are recommended. (See page 43)

17. **True.** Subcutaneous haloperidol can provide effective relief from nausea associated with bowel obstruction. (See page 48)

18. **True.** When mucosal damage contributes to dysphagia, diluted viscous xylocaine can be an effective intervention. (See page 17)

19. **False.** Delirium is very common; up to 85% of terminally ill cancer patients experience this distressing symptom. (See page 56)

20. **True.** When severe, agitated delirium does not respond to other treatments, oral or subcutaneous haloperidol may be the most effective and humane way to control this very distressing symptom. (See page 57)

Posttest

Please read each item and circle the one correct response to each item on the detachable answer sheet at the back of the book.

1. Which of the following is the most important first step when treating non-pain symptoms? (page 6)

[A] Order blood tests and x-rays

[B] Complete a history and physical

[C] Switch the patient's pain medication to an opioid

[D] Order an appropriate adjuvant drug

2. Which of the following nonpain symptoms is least commonly experienced by terminally ill patients? (page 7)

[A] Anorexia

[B] Dyspnea

[C] Nausea

[D] Hiccups

3. Which of the following often contribute to anorexia in the terminally ill? (page 10)

[A] Treatable physical symptoms

[B] Mechanical difficulties with eating

[C] Drug side effects

[D] All of the above

4. Which of the following is an appropriate first step when treating anorexia in an ambulatory terminally ill patient? (page 10)

[A] Order megestrol (Megace) 160-200 mg daily

[B] Order dexamethasone 2-4 mg 1-3 times a day

[C] Assess for presence of oral candidiasis

[D] Order dronabinol (Marinol) 2.5-5.0 mg 2-3 times a day

5. When a terminally ill patient is losing weight due to difficulties with swallowing, which of the following is the most appropriate first step? (page 15)

[A] Surgical resection of the obstructing lesion

[B] Order crushed, liquid, or rectal suppository forms of medication

[C] Placement of an esophageal stent

[D] Palliative radiation therapy

6. When dry mouth is a problem, which of the following is not an appropriate action? (page 16)

[A] Order pilocarpine 5 mg tid

[B] Switch from chlorpromazine (Thorazine) to metoclopramide (Reglan) or haloperidol (Haldol)

[C] Order a saliva substitute q 1-2 hours

[D] Switch from doxepin (Sinequan) to amitriptyline (Elavil)

7. When treating anorexia, which of the following measures is likely to be appropriate in most situations? (page 11)

[A] Patient and family education about the natural progression of cancer and its effects on appetite

[B] Appetite stimulants

[C] IV hydration

[D] Insertion of nasogastric tube

8. When dyspnea is present, which of the following is almost always a factor? (page 27)

[A] Anxiety

[B] Bronchospasm

[C] Low hemoglobin

[D] Airway obstruction

9. When treating dyspnea, which of the following is not appropriate? (page 29)

[A] Reposition the patient to a more upright position

[B] Improve air flow with a fan

[C] Address patient and family anxieties about suffocation

[D] Avoid the use of opioids

10. When treating nonspecific cancer-related dyspnea which of the following is least likely to be an appropriate action? (page 30)

[A] Supportive listening to help relieve anxiety

[B] Thoracentesis to relieve a pleural effusion

[C] Oxycodone 5-10 mg q 4 hours and prn

[D] Naloxone (Narcan) if patient breathes <12/minute

11. When treating cancer-related dyspnea, which of the following classes of drugs is an appropriate first choice? (page 29)

[A] Opioids

[B] Benzodiazepines

[C] Stimulants

[D] Anticholinergics

12. When treating mild dyspnea in patients taking no pain medications, which of the following may be the most appropriate order? (page 29)

   [A] Oxycodone 10 mg q 4 hours and prn
   [B] Acetaminophen with codeine (Tylenol #3) 1 tablet q 4 hours with a booster dose for breakthrough pain of 1 tablet q 2 hours prn
   [C] Hydromorphone (Dilaudid) tablets 2-4 mg q 4 hours with a booster dose for breakthrough pain of 1-2 mg q 2 hours prn
   [D] Slow-release morphine (MS Contin) 30 mg bid

13. Which of the following professionals should be involved in caring for patients with severe dyspnea? (page 26)

   [A] Physician
   [B] Chaplain
   [C] Social Worker
   [D] All of the above

14. When treating severe dyspnea in anxious patients taking strong opioids, which of the following orders may be the most effective? (page 29)

   [A] Hydromorphone (Dilaudid) tablets 1-2 mg q 4 hours and prn and increase dose by 50% q 4-12 hours until relief is achieved
   [B] Acetaminophen with codeine (Tylenol #3) 1 tablet q 4 hours with a booster dose of 1 tablet q 2 hours prn
   [C] Hydrocodone (Hycodan) syrup 1-3 ml q 4 hours with a booster dose of the full 4-hour dose prn
   [D] One hydrocodone (Lortab) tablet 5 mg q 4 hours with a booster dose of 1 tablet q 2 hours prn

15. Which of the following orders is least likely to provide effective relief for patients who are dying of respiratory failure and are experiencing severe dyspnea, anxiety, restlessness, and family stress? (page 31)

   [A] SC infusion of hydromorphone (Dilaudid) with midazolam (Versed) titrated upward until relief achieved
   [B] Chlorpromazine (Thorazine) 25 mg PO or PR q 8 hours
   [C] Phenobarbital 30 mg PO or SC bolus q 8 hours as needed
   [D] Buspirone (Buspar) 5 mg tid

16. Which of the following is least likely to relieve the symptoms of dyspnea? (page 27)

   [A] Companionship
   [B] Isolation
   [C] Spiritual support
   [D] Relaxation

17. Nausea and vomiting usually can be controlled in up to which of the following percentages of patients? (page 40)

   [A] 30%
   [B] 90%
   [C] 10%
   [D] 60%

18. When nausea is the result of increased intracranial pressure, which of the following is the most appropriate treatment? (page 43)

   [A] Dexamethasone
   [B] An antibiotic
   [C] Haloperidol (Haldol)
   [D] Metoclopramide (Reglan)

19. For nausea mediated by the vestibular apparatus, which one of the following is least likely to be an appropriate order? (page 43)

   [A] Meclizine (Antivert)
   [B] Transderm Scop
   [C] Antibiotic and/or decongestant
   [D] Tranquilizers

20. For nausea mediated by the chemoreceptor trigger zone, which one of the following orders is least likely to be effective? (page 43)

   [A] Decrease doses of digoxin and theophylline
   [B] Laxative
   [C] Haloperidol (Haldol) 2 mg PO or SC q 8 hours
   [D] Salt tablets or demeclocycline for low sodium

21. When treating nausea, which of the following are useful measures? (page 41)

   [A] Avoid fatty foods and foods with strong odors
   [B] Serve foods chosen by the patient
   [C] Provide a relaxing atmosphere with pleasant companionship
   [D] All of the above

22. When nausea persists, reassess for which of the following? (page 42)

[A] Bowel obstruction
[B] Drug toxicity
[C] Brain metastases
[D] All of the above

23. When persistent nausea requires the use of subcutaneous antiemetics, which of the following cannot be combined with morphine or hydromorphone (Dilaudid)? (page 45)

[A] Metoclopramide (Reglan)
[B] Hydroxyzine (Vistaril)
[C] Phenytoin (Dilantin)
[D] Haloperidol (Haldol)

24. When severe nausea persists, which of the following medications is least likely to help? (page 45)

[A] Methotrimeprazine (Levoprome) 150 mg/d by SC infusion
[B] Prochlorperazine (Compazine) 5 mg PO or PR tid
[C] Ondansetron (Zofran) 8 mg PO or SC tid
[D] Dexamethasone 4 mg PO or SC bid

25. Symptoms of bowel obstruction include all of the following except which one? (page 46)

[A] Intestinal colic and abdominal pain
[B] Intermittent or continuous vomiting
[C] Urinary retention
[D] Borborygmi (high-pitched bowel sounds)

26. All of the following agents can be used to control the symptoms of bowel obstruction without the use of tubes, diverting surgery, or intravenous fluids, except which one? (page 47)

[A] Analgesics
[B] Bulk laxatives
[C] Anticholinergics
[D] Antiemetics

27. In the hospice/palliative care setting, which of the following interventions is least appropriate to control symptoms associated with bowel obstruction? (page 48)

[A] For pain: Morphine or hydromorphone(Dilaudid) PO, SL, or SC titrated to relief, with the addition of glycopyrrolate (Robinul) 0.4-1.0 m/day SC to relieve cramping pain

[B] For nausea: Haloperidol (Haldol) 5-15 mg/day PO or SC mixed with D5W

[C] For constipation: Docusate 100 mg PO bid-q 4 hours

[D] For anorexia: Nasogastric suction and Ensure 1 can q 4 hours NG or PO

28. When a patient experiences restlessness, which of the following is least likely to be a contributing factor? (page 59)

[A] Pain, low sodium, or high calcium

[B] Hunger or boredom

[C] Fecal impaction or urinary retention

[D] Fear, anxiety, and existential anguish

29. Which of the following is least likely to be an appropriate intervention to relieve restlessness in a terminally ill patient? (page 59)

[A] Supportive counseling to explore psychosocial and spiritual issues

[B] Companionship and distraction activities such as music or reading aloud

[C] Relaxation exercises

[D] Visual imagery of the patient's white blood cells battling tumor cells

30. When no specific cause of restlessness can be identified, which of the following is least likely be an effective order? (page 60)

[A] Lorazepam (Ativan) 0.5-1 mg q 4 hours prn PO or SL

[B] Midazolam (Versed) 2-20 mg per day continuous SC

[C] Haloperidol (Haldol) 5-20 mg per day and midazolam (Versed) 10-100 mg per day continuous SC

[D] Methylphenidate (Ritalin) 10 mg PO tid

31. Delirium is experienced in up to what percentage of terminally ill cancer patients? (page 56)

    [A] 10%
    [B] 30%
    [C] 85%
    [D] 50%

32. Which of the following is not a characteristic of delirium? (page 58)

    [A] Acute onset
    [B] Disorientation and clouding of consciousness
    [C] Impairment of only short-term memory
    [D] Fluctuating course

33. Which of the following is not a common cause of delirium? (page 57)

    [A] Drugs, especially psychotropics
    [B] Falling out of bed
    [C] Stool impaction and urinary tract infections
    [D] Electrolyte or glucose abnormalities

34. When death is approaching and attempts to reverse delirium have been unsuccessful, which of the following is the least appropriate order? (page 57)

    [A] Amitriptyline (Elavil) 20-30 mg IM four times a day and prn
    [B] Haloperidol (Haldol) 1-2 mg PO or SC hourly until calm, then q 6-12 hours
    [C] Thioridazine (Mellaril) 25-50 mg PO hourly until calm then q 6-12 hours
    [D] Chlorpromazine (Thorazine) 25-50 mg PO or PR hourly until calm, then q 6-12 hours

35. For severe agitated delirium, which of the following is the least effective order? (page 57)

    [A] Midazolam (Versed) 0.4-4 mg/hour continuous SC
    [B] Buspirone (Buspar) 5 mg PO hourly prn
    [C] Chlorpromazine (Thorazine) 100 mg every hour IV, PO, or PR
    [D] Methotrimeprazine (Levoprome) 20 mg IM or IV hourly

36. When all other efforts to help relieve severe agitated delirium fail, which of the following is the least appropriate order? (page 58)

   [A] Phenobarbital 130 mg SC hourly until calm and then by subcutaneous infusion (600-1200 mg/day)

   [B] Thiopental (20-200 mg/hr) IV

   [C] Methohexital sodium (Brevital Sodium) continuous IV infusion titrated to relief

   [D] Arm and leg restraints

37. Which of the following is not a benefit of using a portable pump to deliver continuous subcutaneous infusions in the home setting? (page 47)

   [A] Minimal patient discomfort

   [B] It is a simple method for relieving constipation

   [C] Ease of use

   [D] Parenteral administration of combinations of drugs when swallowing is impaired

38. Which of the following is not a common obstacle to the relief of nonpain symptoms? (page 6)

   [A] Family unwillingness to call for help

   [B] Ignoring psychosocial and spiritual aspects of nonpain symptoms

   [C] Physician reluctance to use adequate doses of medications

   [D] Lack of adequate assessment

39. When treating nonpain symptoms in terminally ill patients, which of the following is unnecessary? (page 6)

   [A] Continual reassessment

   [B] Involvement of the entire interdisciplinary team

   [C] Weekly blood counts

   [D] Patient and family education

40. Which of the following is not an effective intervention for dysphagia? (page 14)

   [A] Teaching the family to purée foods

   [B] Treating mucositis with diluted viscous lidocaine

   [C] Emphasizing the family's responsibility to prevent death from starvation

   [D] Treating oral candidiasis with nystatin or ketoconazole

References

[1] Storey P. Symptom control in advanced cancer. *Sem in Onc.* 1994;21(6):748-753.

[2] Bruera E. Research in symptoms other than pain. In: Doyle D, Hanks GWC, MacDonald N, eds. *Oxford Textbook of Palliative Medicine.* New York: Oxford University Press; 1993:87-92.

[3] Portenoy RK, Thaler HT, Kornblith AB, Lepore JM, Friedlander-Klar H, Coyle N, Smart-Curley T, Kemeny N, Norton L, Hoskins W, Scher H. Symptom prevalence, characteristics and distress in a cancer population. *Qual of Life Res.* 1994;3:183-189.

[4] Alexander HR, Norton JA. Pathophysiology of cancer cachexia. In: Doyle D, Hanks GWC, MacDonald N, eds. *Oxford Textbook of Palliative Medicine.* New York: Oxford University Press; 1993:316-329.

[5] Bruera E, Macmillan K, Kuehn N, Hanson J, MacDonald RN. A controlled trial of megestrol acetate on appetite, caloric intake, nutritional status, and other symptoms in patients with advanced cancer. *Cancer.* 1990;66:1279-1282.

[6] Von Roenn JH, Armstrong D, Kotler DP, Cohn DL, Klimas NG, Tchekmedyian NS, Cone L, Brennan PJ, Weitzman SA. Megestrol acetate in patients with AIDS-related cachexia. *Ann Intern Med.* 1994;121:393-399.

[7] Beal JE, Olson R, Laubenstein L, Morales JO, Bellman P, Yangco B, Lefkowitz L, Plasse TF, Shepard KV. Dronabinol as a treatment for anorexia associated with weight loss in patients with AIDS. *J Pain Symptom Manage.* 1995;10(2):89-97.

[8] Terepka AR, Waterhouse C. Metabolic observations during the forced feeding of patients with cancer. *Am J Med.* 1956;225-238.

[9] American College of Physicians. Parenteral nutrition in patients receiving cancer chemotherapy. *Ann Int Med.* 1989;110:734-736.

[10] Kotler DP, Tierney AR, Culpepper-Morgon JA, et al. Effect of home parenteral nutrition on body composition in patients with acquired immunodeficiency syndrome. *J Parenter Enteral Nutr.* 1990;14:454-458.

[11] Burge FI, King DB, Willison D. Intravenous fluids and the hospitalized dying: a medical last rite? *Can Fam Physician.* 1990;36:883-886.

[12] Ciocon JO, Silverstone FA, Graver M, Foley CJ. Tube feedings in elderly patients—indications, benefits, and complications. *Arch Intern Med.* 1988;148:429-433.

[13] Billings, JA. Comfort measures for the terminally ill—is dehydration painful? *J Am Ger Soc.* 1985;33:808-810.

[14] Printz LA. Is withholding hydration a valid comfort measure in the terminally ill? *Geriatrics.* 1988;43:84-88.

References

[15] Andrews MR, Levine AM. Dehydration in the terminal patient: perceptions of hospice nurses. *Am J Hospice Care.* 1989;6:31-34

[16] Terminal dehydration. *Lancet.* 1986;I:306. Editorial.

[17] Miller LJ. Oral pilocarpine for radiation-induced xerostomia. *The Cancer Bulletin.* 1993;45(6):549-550.

[18] Mueller BA, Millheim ET, Farrington EA, Brusko C, Wiser TH. Mucositis management practices for hospitalized patients: national survey results. *J Pain Symptom Manage.* 1995;10(7):510-520.

[19] Ellershaw JE, Sutcliffe JM, Saunders CM. Dehydration and the dying patient. *J Pain Symptom Manage.* 1995;10(3):192-197.

[20] Ahmedzai S. Palliation of respiratory symptoms. In: Doyle D, Hanks GWC, MacDonald N, eds. *Oxford Textbook of Palliative Medicine.* New York: Oxford University Press; 1993:349-378.

[21] Gleeson C, Spencer D. Blood transfusion and its benefits in palliative care. *Palliat Med.* 1995;9:307-231.

[22] Bruera E, MacEachern T, Ripamonti C, Hanson J. Subcutaneous morphine for dyspnea in cancer patients. *Ann Intern Med.* 1993;119:906-907.

[23] Light RW, Muro JR, Sato RI, Stansbury DW, Fischer CE, Brown SE. Effects of oral morphine on breathlessness and exercise tolerance in patients with chronic obstructive pulmonary disease. *Am Rev Respir Dis.* 1989;139:126-133.

[24] Bottomley DM, Hanks GW. Subcutaneous midazolam infusion in palliative care. *J Pain Symptom Manage.* 1990;5:259-261.

[25] Reuben DB, Morch V. Nausea and vomiting in terminal cancer patients. *Arch Inter Med.* 1986;146:2021-2023.

[26] Lichter I. Results of antiemetic management in terminal illness. *J Palliat Care.* 1993;9:19-21.

[27] Baines M, Oliver DJ, Carter RL. Medical management of intestinal obstruction in patients with advanced malignant disease—a clinical and pathological study. *Lancet.* 1985;2:990-993.

[28] Ripamonti C, Conno FD, Ventafridda V, Rossi B, Baines MJ. Management of bowel obstruction in advanced and terminal cancer patients. *Ann Onc.* 1993;4:15-21.

[29] Storey P, Hill HH, St. Louis RH, Tarver EE. Subcutaneous infusions for control of cancer symptoms. *J Pain Symptom Manage.* 1990;5:33-41.

[30] Oliver DJ. The use of methotrimeprazine in terminal care. *Br J Cli Pract.* 1985;22:339-340.

[31] Mulvenna PM, Regnard CFB. Subcutaneous ondansetron. *Lancet.* 1992;339:1059.

[32] Tunca JC, Buchler DA, Mack EA, Ruzicka FF, Crowley JJ, Carr WF. The management of ovarian-cancer-caused bowel obstruction. *Gynecol Onc.* 1981;12:186-192.

[33] Lund B, Hansen M, Lundvall F, Nielsen NC, Sorenson BL, Hansen HH. Intestinal obstruction in patients with advanced carcinoma of the ovaries treated with combination chemotherapy. *Surg Gynecol Obstet.* 1989;169:213-218.

[34] Mercadante S, Spoldi E, Caraceni A, Maddaloni S, Simonetti MT. Ocetreotide in relieving gastrointestinal symptoms due to bowel obstruction. *Pall Med.* 1993;7:295-299.

[35] Breitbart W, Bruera E, Chochinov H, Lynch M. Neuropsychiatric syndromes and psychological symptoms in patients with advanced cancer. *J Pain Symptom Manage.* 1995;10(2):131-141.

[36] Fainsinger R, Bruera E. The management of dehydration in terminally ill patients. *J Palliat Care.* 1994;10(3):55-59.

[37] Bruera E, Miller L, McCallion J, Macmillan K, Krefting L, Hanson J. Cognitive failure in patients with terminal cancer: a prospective study. *J Pain Symptom Manage.* 1992;7:192-195.

[38] Twycross RG, Lichter I. The terminal phase. In: Doyle D, Hanks GW, MacDonald N, eds. *Oxford Textbook of Palliative Medicine.* New York: Oxford University Press; 1993:651-661.

[39] Greene WR, Davis WH. Titrated intravenous barbiturates in the control of symptoms in patients with terminal cancer. *South Med J.* 1991;84:332-337.

[40] Truog RD, Berde CB, Mitchell C, Grier HE. Barbiturates in the care of the terminally ill. *N Engl J Med.* 1992;327:1678-82.

[41] Cherny NI, Coyle N, Foley KM. The treatment of suffering when patients request elective death. *J Palliat Care.* 1994;10(2):71-79.

Notes

Posttest Answer Sheet

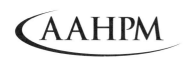

UNIPAC Four: Management of Selected Nonpain Symptoms in the Terminally Ill

Physicians are eligible to receive 3 credit hours in Category 1 of the AMA/PRA by completing and returning this posttest answer sheet to the AAHPM. The Academy will keep a record of AMA/PRA Category 1 credit hours and the record will be provided on request; however, physicians are responsible for reporting their own Category 1 CME credits when applying for the AMA/PRA or for other certificates or credentials.

Name

Street

City/State/Zip Code

Telephone

Social Security Number

Please mail this answer sheet and a check payable to *"AAHPM"* in the amount of:

$45.00 — *AAHPM members*
$60.00 — *non-members*

Physician Training Programs
American Academy of Hospice
  and Palliative Medicine
PO Box 14288
Gainesville, FL 32604-2288

Please circle the one correct answer for each question.

1.	A	B	C	D	15.	A	B	C	D	29.	A B C D
2.	A	B	C	D	16.	A	B	C	D	30.	A B C D
3.	A	B	C	D	17.	A	B	C	D	31.	A B C D
4.	A	B	C	D	18.	A	B	C	D	32.	A B C D
5.	A	B	C	D	19.	A	B	C	D	33.	A B C D
6.	A	B	C	D	20.	A	B	C	D	34.	A B C D
7.	A	B	C	D	21.	A	B	C	D	35.	A B C D
8.	A	B	C	D	22.	A	B	C	D	36.	A B C D
9.	A	B	C	D	23.	A	B	C	D	37.	A B C D
10.	A	B	C	D	24.	A	B	C	D	38.	A B C D
11.	A	B	C	D	25.	A	B	C	D	39.	A B C D
12.	A	B	C	D	26.	A	B	C	D	40.	A B C D
13.	A	B	C	D	27.	A	B	C	D		
14.	A	B	C	D	28.	A	B	C	D		

Notes

Notes

… Notes

Notes

Notes

Notes

Notes